Virtuous Transcendence

Holistic Self-Cultivation and Self-Healing in Elderly Korean Immigrants

HAWORTH Aging, Psychology, and Mental Health
T. L. Brink, PhD
Senior Editor

A Guide to Psychological Practice in Geriatric Long-Term Care by Peter A. Lichtenberg

Mental Health Practice in Geriatric Health Care Settings by Peter A. Lichtenberg

Virtuous Transcendence: Holistic Self-Cultivation and Self-Healing in Elderly Korean Immigrants by Keum Young Chung Pang

Virtuous Transcendence

Holistic Self-Cultivation and Self-Healing in Elderly Korean Immigrants

Keum Young Chung Pang

The Haworth Press®
New York • London • Oxford

The Haworth Press, Inc., 10 Alice Street, Binghamton, NY 13904-1580

Cover design by Marylouise Doyle.

Library of Congress Cataloging-in-Publication Data

Pang, Keum Young Chung.

Virtuous transcendence: holistic self-cultivation and self-healing in elderly Korean immigrants / Keum Y. Pang.

p. cm.

Includes bibliographical references and index.

ISBN 0-7890-0928-5 (hard)—ISBN 0-7890-0929-3 (pbk.)

1. Korean Americans—Health and hygiene—United States. 2. Immigrants—Health and hygiene—United States. 3. Aged—Health and hygiene—United States. 4. Health attitudes—United States. 5. Aged—Cross-cultural studies I. Title.

RA418.5T73 P36 2000
613'.089'957073—dc21 99-055442

CONTENTS

ABOUT THE AUTHOR

Medical anthropologist **Keum Young Chung Pang, PhD, RN** is Professor at Howard University in Washington, DC. She was born in Korea and educated there as well as in England and the United States. Before she came to Howard University, she taught at the Catholic University of America in Washington, DC, and Niagara University. Dr. Pang had a joint teaching appointment at the College of Medicine, Howard University, to work with psychiatric residents for transcultural mental health care. She has conducted funded research projects including the study "Depression, Somatization, and Korean Elderly Immigrants." Her research funds were granted by the National Institute of Aging, NIH, U.S. Public Health Service, and the Howard University Faculty Research Support Grant. Dr. Pang is the author of *Korean Elderly Women in America* and has published numerous papers in nationally and internationally peer-reviewed scholarly journals. She is the recipient of a National Research Service Award and British Council Fellowship, and served on the Planning Committee of the International Council of Nurses (ICN) in 1987.

Foreword

Reading through this collection of life stories of Korean elders, drawn from a study of depression among members of this community, is at first disorienting. The narratives that emerge are not organized around the classic diagnostic criteria of depressive illness, nor around categories that form the basis for most epidemiological studies today—symptoms, care-seeking practices, medications used and their efficacy, social networks, social support, or social functioning. Instead, one is introduced into lifeworlds of suffering, lifeworlds of elderly men and women who have lived through extraordinary times, and men and women who reside in the United States but are still deeply invested in Korean historical memories and values. Furthermore, the reader often finds it difficult to distinguish those who meet criteria for depression from those who do not. Rather than providing neat evidence for either a universal or more cultural understanding of depressive illness, these narratives raise more fundamental questions about the appropriateness of a taken-for-granted view of depression as illness. The cumulative effect of reading through these life stories, one after another, is a growing understanding of a civilization, a historical trajectory of a people, and ways that individuals and families attempt to respond to massive calamites and personal tragedies—to what Arthur Kleinman calls "social suffering" (Kleinman, Das, and Lock, 1996).

The book consists not of grand themes or theoretical speculations, but of bits of data from interviews with one after another elderly Korean man and woman. Classic problems of older Americans, as well as problems particular to elders displaced to new societies and separated from the sounds and smells and tastes of their earlier lives, are present in the details of these conversations. Struggles with language, frustration over transportation difficulties, a sense of social isolation and loss of access to old friendships, and a more basic sense of loss of the everyday lifeworld of Korean society emerge in the complaints voiced by these men and women. More distinctive aspects of the lives of Korean elders emerge as well. Historical memories of suffering and deprivation associated with the Japanese occupation and the great Korean war betray the hidden scars as well as the great strength of these survivors. The stories of these elders point over and over again to the deep, enduring civilizational values focused on generational relations—on the value that accrues in sacrificing for one's children, on "filial piety" and the care elders expect from their children, and on the joys and disappointments of relations with children and grandchildren as one ages. These generational values and the conflicts that emerge from them are revealed, at the same time, as deeply patriarchal. The elder women remember lives with mothers-in-law, and later with daughters-in-law, and one has a sense that relations among women are devalued and complicated by values of patriarchy. An elder woman's desire to live with her son, rather than her daughter, places her in a conflicted field with both her daughter and her son's wife. For any who might romanticize "Eastern" or Asian cultures, thinking that norms of filial piety and respect for elders removes the sting of aging, reading these stories will be instructive. Norms of filial piety lead to hopes and expectations that can never be fully met in old age, just as values of independence lead to hopes and expectations that can never be realized by aging Americans.

At the same time, the life stories presented here provide a picture of elders attempting to achieve a distinctively Korean form of equanimity—a sense of balance, harmony, peace, human compassion, dignity—produced self-consciously through practices of self-cultivation. These practices are embodied, affecting the vital organs and producing harmonious functioning, just as chaotic thoughts, anger, and emotional distress are linked to chaotic, depleted, shrunken or swollen vital organs, resulting in bodily distress and named conditions such as *hwabyung* or *shingyungshayak.* But even these so-called culture-bound disorders or popular illness categories are ambiguous, as revealed in these pages. Though denoting embodied distress, they are at the same time badges of honor, a symbol of perserverance, "symptoms" of the sacrifices and suffering endured throughout a lifetime. They also point to a more fundamental vision in Korean society of the deeply tragic dimensions of the human condition, of history, and of society. There is no easy optimism in these stories, no simple sense that life should be free of pain or sadness and that one deserves happiness and comfort as the culmination of life. None of this suggests that there is no depression among Korean elders, or that medical or mental health interventions are inappropriate. One might argue quite the opposite. But it does make clear that any sense that cultural difference resides simply in slight variations in symptom expression or duration criteria misses the point of the anthropological vision. What we learn from these Korean elders and the stories that they tell, as well as from Dr. Pang's editing, arranging and analysis of them, is that the pain of living leaves marks that are not simply symptoms of an illness, but memorials of perserverance, embodied signs of social suffering, and marks of the human condition. It is a lesson not easy to assimilate.

Byron J. Good
Department of Social Medicine
Harvard Medical School

REFERENCE

Arthur Kleinman, Veena Das, and Margaret Lock, eds. *Social Suffering*. Daedalus, Winter 1996.

NOTES FOR PROFESSIONAL LIBRARIANS AND LIBRARY USERS

This is an original book title published by The Haworth Press, Inc. Unless otherwise noted in specific chapters with attribution, materials in this book have not been previously published elsewhere in any format or language.

CONSERVATION AND PRESERVATION NOTES

All books published by The Haworth Press, Inc. and its imprints are printed on certified ph neutral, acid free book grade paper. This paper meets the minimum requirements of American National Standard for Information Sciences-Permanence of Paper for Printed Material, ANSI Z39.48-1984.

Preface

Through my in-depth research, I have gathered and interpreted elderly Korean immigrants' personal stories about their everyday lives, illnesses, and self-care methods in an American and Korean context. In this book, I discuss the origin and phenomenology of illness in the elderly. The dominant themes are their self-care patterns, reconciliation, spiritualism, and transcendence. I present the original and revolutionary idea of somatization as a self-care process. Using a rigorous research method to identify relevant observed behaviors, I attempt to clarify the interrelationships among anger, depression, Korean popular illnesses such as *hwabyung,* and somatization-psychologization. The relationships have been unclear until now despite decades of study. The relationship between mind and body has been studied in the context of social structure, cosmology, energy, and language, as well as cognitive and visual modes of symptom expression. However, this study is unique, with fresh new ways of looking at and thinking about the holistic perspective on human conditions. It is a culturally vivid work. The narratives themselves will touch every reader's heart. Here is an opportunity to truly appreciate the subtlety and delicacy of Korean ethnography. Harmoniously interwoven in this tapestry of rich and vivid stories is a blend of proverbs, cultural analysis, and scholarly and empathetic interpretation. This book will help readers understand why elderly Korean immigrants behave holistically!

I am a Korean American. I have lived half of my life in Korea and the other half in America. I could be considered an insider as well as an outsider in both of these countries. With my personal background and scholarly ability, I am able to balance both emic and etic perspectives. I gently embrace the experience of illness as a holistic biopsychological and sociocultural self-healing phenomenon. I show in detail how human beings work toward harmony when East meets West. The Korean cultural current is subtle yet clearly reflected in their efforts toward acculturation. This book presents a blend of theory, research, and self-healing practices in everyday life. In addition, this paradigm can effectively stimulate the combination of research and theory, which may help in reaching therapeutic goals among other ethnic populations.

As we live in a time of global culture, it seems vital to understand how people become ill and how they get better. This book is also about older adults, who are increasing in number. We live in a time of holistic, pluralistic, and spiritual therapeutic choices. The public is aware of the need to examine new explanatory models with which they are not familiar. But the message in this book can be applied to people of most ages. This volume addresses how we can understand and interpret our emotional climate and apply self-care. The model described offers a different avenue for self-care by generating harmony within the individual and by sharing with others for harmonious interpersonal relationships and happiness, especially for people who are culturally and ethnically different.

The purpose of this book is to assist laypeople and health providers in understanding the cultural differences and similarities faced by elderly Korean immigrants living in the United States. Elderly Korean immigrants experience everyday life stresses such as marginalization with sociocultural differences, intergenerational differences, lack of freedom, inevitable dependent living, financial problems, health problems, role loss, loss of loved ones, ambivalent relationships with children, facing their own deaths, and so on. These phenomena may make elderly Koreans depressed and cause them to suffer from popular illnesses such as *han, hwabyung,* or *shingyungshayak.* Sometimes these conditions cause physical ailments such as heart disease, hypertension, indigestion, and so on. Some of the informants were diagnosed with major depression. However, they have not been hospitalized, nor have they been taking antidepressants. Apparently, they have been helping themselves in some way.

Self-care and self-healing originate from self-cultivation. According to Korean beliefs, a person becomes self-cultivated when he or she exchanges compassion (*chong*) with others in a mature fashion. The individual overcomes fate instead of succumbing to it. The self-cultivated person controls anger. He or she maintains peace of mind and thus is not stirred easily. He or she is self-disciplined, promoting and maintaining equanimity. The person is healthy, stable, and wise.

Self-cultivated people do not allow themselves to suffer from depression, *han, hwabyung,* or *shingyungshayak,* the latter three of which are referred to as Korean popular illnesses. If they have these kinds of problems, they can get rid of them as they become self-cultivated and self-disciplined. Usually, the healing process begins by telling a story (i.e., using an explanatory model and semantic networks) behind one or more of the illnesses to sympathetic listeners. As a result, the sufferers can develop insight into themselves and their problems. They are able to get to know themselves better and resolve their problems by changing undesirable behaviors into desirable ones. Others may give them support as it is needed.

One informant said, "I think I am getting wise as I am getting older. Now I can enjoy my life as it is and I even can appreciate how valuable my life is. I am able to accept myself as I am, what I do, and everything as it is." As they mature and become wise, they relax, feeling less fear of making mistakes and bringing shame to themselves and others. Korean elders may resolve conflicts through *ch'enyom,* a right way of thinking. Other disciplined ways of self-healing include physical exercise, hygiene, nutrition, religion, and recreation, such as music. The combination of mind-body self-care and healing methods generates vital energy for a healthy mind and body.

I would like to acknowledge with gratitude the support of the National Institute of Aging, Howard University Faculty Support Grant, Amerasian Data Research Services, and a Northeast Asia Council Research Grant. I would like to express my gratitude to our elderly Korean immigrant informants. Their loving, smiling faces make a panorama in my memory. I thank Dean Warren K. Ashe, Professor Won Sul Lee, and Dr. Man Yul Lee for their invaluable suggestions for my research. I am very grateful indeed to Professor Byron J. Good for his priceless advice and guidance on my research, publications, scholarly work, and professional development over a decade. I am indebted to Professor Arthur Kleinman for his theoretical emphasis. I acknowledge with gratitude the critical reading of the manuscript by Dr. Emeline Otey. I wish to thank Professor T. Brink, Senior Editor of Haworth's Aging, Psychology, and

Mental Health book program, and the anonymous reviewers. I am very thankful to Anna Buc for putting this book together enthusiastically with her special editorial and computer knowledge and skills. She painstakingly read the manuscript numerous times and corrected and rewrote again and again. I would like to thank Helen Sirkin and Irene Marsh, who took time from their busy schedules to offer editorial assistance. This book could not have been written without understanding, encouragement, and direct assistance from my parents, husband, Sunjoo Pang, and son, David Sooho Pang. I am truly indebted to them.

Keum Young Chung Pang
Washington, DC

Introduction

This text was integrated and interpreted with the review of old and new literature in Korean and English. The literature included Korean culture, history, religion, medicine, healing, self-care, social sciences, and cross-cultural studies of depression; Korean elderly immigrants' explanatory models; semantic networks; Korean popular illness and idioms; and Korean proverbs in their cultural context. As a medical anthropologist and a community psychiatric mental health nurse, I studied everyday life, depression, somatization, Korean popular illnesses, and the self-care of elderly Korean immigrants in the Washington, DC, metropolitan area. The National Institute on Aging (NIA) supported this research from 1991 to 1996.

The findings of this study may apply to other East Asians, particularly Chinese and Japanese immigrants, because of the similarities in value orientation and cognitive emotional aspects. They share Confucianism and other similar cultural and religious influences. For example, Chinese, Japanese, and Koreans suffer from neurasthenia. When I was discussing my research as a guest lecturer at the Catholic University of America in Washington, DC, in April 1997, a doctoral student from mainland China in the ethnopsychology class said, "Everything that you lectured and wrote in your articles is the same as in my country." The paradigm of relating depression to Korean folk or popular illnesses in my research could be applied to other ethnic populations, particularly East Asians who are influenced by Confucianism, with some modifications. Also, this research may be helpful in understanding Western depression and other illness behaviors more broadly and deeply through comparison and contrast.

A young second-generation Korean-American man asked, "Why are all Korean things sad?" That was his overall perception of Korean art, such as movies and songs. Koreans tend to sentimentalize and romanticize even casual meetings or partings in comparison to Americans and seem to appreciate the melancholy of a sentimental nature, probably because they have faced sad events and circumstances: human cruelty, tragedy, hunger and poverty, lack of educational opportunity, death, separation from loved ones by wars, rejection, betrayal, and mistrust by loved ones, to mention some examples. They might have developed certain ways of turning depression into a kind of sweet sorrow to be able to live with it instead of abhorring it.

Korean elders are traditionally cared for by their children. However, some Korean immigrant elders now live by themselves, longing for human caring and warmth. Others are quite happy being alone. By presenting selected stories of older Korean men and women, their contented times, fun times, difficult times, sad, depressed, betrayed, or rejected times, respected times, and hopeful times will be reflected. The reader can learn about their life patterns, values, beliefs, attitudes, and even personalities. Their stories include their present and past experiences in America and Korea. I have included their own narratives to share these experiences directly, instead of using watered-down reports by third persons.

The stories told by older Korean immigrants have similarities and differences, which may be subtle or drastic. Although the stories all seem to be the same in a broad sense, because they are all related to individual Korean experiences, customs, and views of the world, differences and similarities appear in expressing daily life, illnesses, and self-care experiences according to their biopsychosocial conditions, emotions, and beliefs.

Are elderly Korean immigrants really depressed? What kinds of problems do they have? How do they solve them? What do they think of their everyday life situations? How well do they live by themselves and with their children? What are the ways they express their distress? What idioms do they use to express their feelings and thoughts?

I will introduce various life patterns by presenting each elder's unique experience. My wish is to present the Korean elders' souls, minds, and emotions in their stories as they told them, and to show how they expressed them as accurately as possible so that readers can look deep into the elders' hearts to understand who they are, what they do, and what they think. As much as possible, I want to avoid the risk of inadvertently altering their true meanings and intended messages by curtailing the natural flow of their life's experiences. When each Korean elder's information is presented, a brief sociodemographic background is provided. For the sake of organization, I have arranged the text into two parts: ethos, health, and illness in Part I; and Korean-American stories with interpretations and analysis in Part II. An epilogue includes a discussion and conclusion; it is followed by a glossary, bibliography, and index. The ten chapters are related to Korean elders' major concerns and interests, such as the lives of immigrants, family, children, marriage, health, illness, self-help, and death. Their stories will be interpreted, as appropriate, in an American and Korean context analytically as well as synthetically, as much as possible, because life experiences occur holistically and synchronously. This way, some indirect suggestions for holistic community health policy as well as holistic biopsychosocial and cultural explanatory models and semantic networks may emerge for effective health service. The stories might help us understand how Koreans construct and deconstruct their popular illnesses, depression, and relationships.

THEORETICAL FOUNDATION

The importance of storytelling is in the truly healing process that comes through reminiscences, self-knowledge, self-awareness, and a form of catharsis. It is very important to talk to a confidant about problems. In this book, the cross-cultural concerns and phenomena of the study of depression are pointed out generally and specifically in Korean explanatory models and semantic networks. The literature related to cultural forces and their influence on understanding depression was reviewed to learn what and how depression-related phenomena are expressed. Korean popular illnesses—*hwabyung* (physical and emotional distress with complaints of having a lump in the throat or abdomen, which may cause feelings of pain, indigestion, or suffocation), *han* (passive expression of regrets and resentment with complaints of a lump at times), and *shingyung-shayak* (neurasthenia, psychoneurotically based physical and emotional syndromes)—are introduced in Chapter 1 in relation to life stress, anger, depressed mood, and illness behaviors in the Korean cultural context. I discuss the psychodynamics of dysphoria in Koreans in terms of demoralization with interpersonal disharmony. The following are some of the examples I reviewed for the theoretical foundations of the cross-cultural study of depression in Koreans: Lin (1983) (*hwabyung* as a culture-bound syndrome), Kuo (1984) (Korean immigrants' high depression rate), and the related literature initiated by American authors such as Arthur Kleinman (1995) (rethinking of somatization), Byron Good (1977) (semantic networks), Good and Good (1981) (semantic networks), as well as Korean authors such as Bou Yong Rhi (1983 and 1986) (Koreans' tendency of somatization) and Kwang Iel Kim (1991) (cross-cultural psychiatry and care). Explanatory models and semantic networks have been integral and instrumental in developing the strategy for cross-cultural interpretation.

Included are Korean illnesses related to depression; body-mind-nature-related self-cultivation; Korean traditional medical reality; pluralistic religious backgrounds; historical, economical, and political influences; conceptualizations of ancestors, filial piety, marriage, children, and family; Korean proverbs related to everyday life; self-care beliefs and practices; relationships with children; and conditions of immigration. All of these are needed to illustrate the Korean cultural background necessary to discuss the construction of illness.

Korean idioms used for anger, depression, and sadness are dealt with extensively in explanatory models and semantic networks in this book. Some examples given in the text are related to a son's alcoholism, a husband's indifference, and a daughter's betrayal. First, the related stories are presented, and then they are analyzed and interpreted holistically. Korean illness idioms become catalysts for catharsis and ultimately healing. So we see that Korean illnesses have multiple beneficial roles as well as illness roles. It sounds paradoxical! But it seems to be true.

The relationship between psychologization and somatization in symptom presentation is reflected in this study. The notion that psychologization occurs in certain cultures such as that of the West, while somatization occurs in certain others such as the Chinese (Kleinman, 1980) has been a controversial one. Later, Kleinman (1995) addresses it as more interrelated, systematic, holistic experiences. Here, personality, intimacy, and confidant relationships are reviewed in relation to dysphoria and its alleviation and prevention. Also dealt with are the Korean emotional climate and moral and ethical issues.

The impact of family and social structural changes—from nuclear family to extended family and from individualism to collectivism—on interactions between parents and children was examined. Korean social structure has been discussed as a system that requires alternative communication patterns in the expression of illness for healing by using the idioms of Korean illness. Multireligious, syncretic backgrounds with shamanism, Buddhism, Confucianism, and Christianity have been looked at in regard to the prevalent spiritual healing of anger and depression-related illnesses.

Healing behaviors were reviewed, including the Korean emotional and behavioral holistic ethos:

1. *Chong*—behaviors and attitudes that originate, create, and emanate compassionate relationships
2. *Fate*—an alternative motivating and empowering force
3. *Ch'enyom*—transcendental resolution of distressing worldly affairs through self-care
4. *Tchang*—singing, usually agonized, sad Korean folk songs with special cathartic and meditative vocalization of regrets, resentments, and transcendence for holistic healing
5. *Moo*—Korean folk dancing, usually expressing sad and transcending moods, with special cathartic and meditative movements representing regrets, resentment, and, finally, transcendence for holistic healing
6. Similar exercises for obtaining vital energy

METHOD

Chapter 2 describes the use of the Korean Depression Interview Schedule (KDIS-III), the Semistructured Korean Interview Guide for Depression (SKIGD), the sampling method, and the directions for analysis and interpretation of the narratives, as well as a brief sociodemographic discussion of the elderly Korean immigrants in the study.

We interviewed 674 Korean older adults using KDIS-III, modified with Korean cultural considerations, and screened thirty-five informants who had experienced major depression sometime in their lives. We interviewed thirty-four of these informants with depression, and thirty-five without depression, with the SKIGD, which was constructed by the author. SKIGD contains questions about the experiences of old age, living conditions in Korea and America, sadness and depression, Korean popular illnesses (*hwabyung, han,* and *shingyung-shayak*), and the relationship between depression and Korean illnesses and healing behaviors, especially self-care. Some anger pervades the immigrants' narratives as they try to "melt away" or "digest" their illnesses with traditional self-care methods.

The informants told their stories about their lives and illnesses in terms of why they had or did not have anger, sorrow, or depression; what their life conditions were like; understanding their illnesses and symptoms; how they felt about having or not having depression or Korean popular illnesses; and how they managed their experiences.

TRYING TO LIVE AS AMERICANS DO

The Korean informants told their life stories relating to both joyful and stressful experiences in the acculturation process. Sometimes euphoric, optimistic, and ambitious, yet ambivalent, immigrant lives unfolded in these stories, which are presented in Chapter 3. Their emotional climate fluctuated between exultation and despair as they faced life events. Such events included unexpected actions by the American government (changes in housing and monthly monetary assistance), conflict with children over cultural and intergenerational differences, experiences of discrimination, and stress while helping children to adjust and preparing for the citizenship test at the same time. Most of the informants found the welfare system in the United States a pleasant surprise. Among elderly Korean immigrants there seems to be a correlation between independence from their children and contentment with themselves and their children. The elderly Koreans tried not to interfere with their children's efforts for a successful immigrant life, or with their health and welfare. In the majority of cases, the parents made sacrifices for their children. They experienced the phenomena of becoming aware of, responding to, learning, and practicing living in a multiethnic environment. Racial discrimination and difficult low-wage jobs were a reality for the immigrants.

STILL LIVING BY KOREAN CUSTOMS

The cultural workings of Korean values and beliefs are expressed, expected, practiced, encouraged, and sometimes resisted by elderly Korean immigrants and their children. *Hwabyung,* a Korean popular illness, is experienced if Koreans resist the formal observance of ancestor veneration ceremonies. Submissiveness and obedience are highly valued. Contentment with harsh living conditions is believed to be a virtue in Korean culture. Causes of depression or illness could include, for instance, the loss of one's image as a wise mother and a good wife. The perception of appearing uncultivated, the stresses of the four-generation family, the strain of being old but continuing to work—all are factors that could cause illness. Talking, understanding, and obtaining resolution is healing. Health maintenance and promotion are explained in terms of religious, spiritual, self-cultivated attitudes and behaviors in dealing with conflicts. Culture-specific illness does not seem to be prevalent among elders near or over eighty years old, because these informants seem to be less concerned about matters such as interpersonal and health issues.

PARENTS CAN TAKE CARE OF TEN CHILDREN, BUT TEN CHILDREN CANNOT SUPPORT THEIR PARENTS

Korean elders' choices about whether to live with their children, along with stories about children's deaths, sorrow, and its transcendence are described and interpreted in Chapter 5. Some informants are satisfied with their relationships with their children. Intergenerational conflicts with their children and grandchildren in relation to financial dealings, reactions to conditional reciprocal relationships, perceptions of lack of caring and support, and disease and illness constructions related to distress are included. Korean parents do not always perceive their children as devoted, but parents take care of their children as much as they can no matter how old the parents and their children are. The comedies and tragedies of the ambivalence in parent-child relationships emerge as the elders are inevitably dependent upon their children, despite their best efforts to be independent in their acculturation process. The struggles caused by the change from Korean traditional values to values in America are discussed. The construction of illness based on reality as influenced by past conditions, the acculturation process, holistic healing, cognitive emotional phenomena, and other health behaviors are studied. The elderly Koreans' separation anxiety due to the painful experience of acculturation is often expressed.

FAMILY LIFE

Chapter 6 describes the informants' perceptions of their children's situations, their relationships with other children, and the elders' endeavors to smooth the frictions in relationships with their children by using self-cultivation—Korean ways of making peace with others and themselves. With self-help, they reduce their children's burdens by understanding and assisting them as much as they can, even when it causes enormous inconvenience and requires sacrifices in their own lives. Most of the time, the parents' anguish and sadness are melted away by their children's filial care. On the other hand, an elderly mother expressed intolerance regarding her adult son's burden of household chores, traditionally considered women's tasks, assigned to him by his wife (her daughter-in-law). Elderly Koreans face difficulty in accepting societal changes in gender roles reflected in the family. Intergenerational conflicts are frequently encountered. Also, the shameful and guilty feelings aroused by the deaths of a spouse or children in the Korean context are presented and interpreted.

WOMEN'S LIVES

Chapter 7 mainly depicts unfortunate marital experiences. An informant was able to forgive her "unforgivable husband" by God's grace and now enjoys peace of mind. Another informant is still experiencing the residual effects of spousal abuse. The physical and psychological abuse of another wife is narrated and interpreted. Agony and distress tend to be expressed as a combination of physical, emotional, and mental phenomena. Scenes of enduring marital discourse and protecting oneself from inner injury by assuming an attitude of internal superiority are discussed. The informants use the idioms of Korean popular illness for expressing their cognitive, emotional, and physical phenomena to promote healing in the Korean familiar paradigm. In this way they are able to understand the problems in their lives and resolve them. The dual roles of Korean illnesses have been discussed: illness and the healing process. The emotional distress and inner spiritual wounds of the Korean elders are healed by their self-acceptance, acceptance of the reality around them, and by understanding human nature through spiritual and religious awakening. The appreciation of nature, music, art such as calligraphy, and physical exercise contribute to this healing process.

The fear of death in terms of phenomena and process was expressed. Some regretted that they did not do much for people other than themselves and their family. Informants who are familiar with Western medicine do not seem to rely on Korean self-healing processes. Some alternative ways of self-healing from the trauma of a husband's extramarital affairs are revealed.

MEN'S LIVES

Loneliness is the main concern of Korean men. However, some informants create ways to spend their time meaningfully every day. Sometimes they appear vulnerable yet resilient. Their moods fluctuate according to their everyday life problems: conflicts with children in terms of communication and value differences, health problems, self-esteem, financial problems, or perceiving life to be meaningless. Assuming responsibility for household chores that were traditionally considered women's work affects men's self-esteem. An informant said, "I have to cook and wash although I am an old man. Can you imagine that?"

In Chapter 8, an elderly Korean man shares his experiences and the meaning of his unhappy marriage and lonely widower's life. Another elderly man is learning that his children's support is not given if parental duty and responsibility have not been fulfilled first.

HEALTH, ILLNESS, AND SELF-CARE

The phenomena of health, illness, and self-healing among Koreans are described in Chapter 9. The expressions of their emotional distress in relation to their children, spouses, and their hardships are depicted at times by using the idioms of Korean illnesses such as *hwabyung*. The objective nature of the phenomenon of depression is claimed to change according to psychosocial situations. Symptomatologically and phenomenologically, emotion is managed as a unique individual experience with a variety of expressions. It is believed that mental agony is associated with commonly diagnosed physical diseases. Preventive and self-care methods with high moral standards of conduct through self-cultivation, religious faith, syncretic healing patterns, spiritual inner strength, transition from active work to spiritual devotion in retirement as a prevention, and nature-oriented physical activities based on Korean value orientations are described. Although it may sound paradoxical, the construction of illnesses ultimately seems to deconstruct the illnesses. The prevention and healing of illnesses among these Korean informants is often accomplished by discussing one's symptoms in terms of one or more Korean illnesses and then through self-resolution of conflicts and holistic self-healing.

The will of the human being in nature is considered the essence of self-help and healing. Thus, almost every informant in our research says, "Medications do not work." It is considered lucky to have devoted children not only for their support but also, even more important, because the very thought of having caring children makes elders reassured and content to be healthy. "Let us be free and independent, let us live courageously and patiently, and cultivate ourselves to be healthy" is a loud message from the informants. Another message is to redirect life, turn negative thinking into positive, and strengthen spirituality to be healthy and happy. The informants tend to positively use a cognition oriented to God's will for transcending undesirable life events.

AT LAST, DEATH

What are Koreans' thoughts and attitudes in dealing with the last rite, death? Some elderly Koreans, particularly those around ninety years of age, said that they are genuinely ready to relinquish their lives naturally and leave this world for another without ambivalence or even any sense of attachment or regret. They have already nearly transcended this world. Still, they perceive their future death and the dying process as extraordinary phenomena.

Koreans seem to be comfortable with death even though they have not prepared, in a worldly sense, for the last rite, with the exception of some decisions such as choosing the clothes to be worn when they are buried. There is no discussion with their children about the funeral, for example. This may be because of their traditional extended family living and multiple religious influences. Their philosophy of life appears to be that one should not overdo anything but wait for nature to take care of things. Their attitude is, "Don't worry, somehow it will be taken care of. Most things in the world have been that way and so it will be."

THEORETICAL BACKGROUND IN SOMATIZATION AND SELF-CARE

The ultimate purpose of this book is to elicit and interpret the ethos of elderly Korean immigrants as reflected in their everyday lives and their health and illness beliefs and practices. The whole person, or a group of people, can be understood through their depressed, difficult, frustrated, and sad life experiences.

The author constructed the Semistructured Korean Interview Guide for Depression (SKIGD), which contains open-ended questions to elicit Korean elderly immigrants' narratives including their spontaneous feelings and thoughts about their current lives, life situations in Korea before immigration, immigrant lives, sadness and depression, and experiences with culture-specific illnesses. The approaches of explanatory models and semantic networks were used for data collection, analysis, and interpretation in the Korean cultural context. The seventy Korean informants selected, except for one case, were interviewed with SKIGD. Forty-one stories out of sixty-nine were selected for this book to avoid repetition of similar themes.

The elderly Korean immigrants' life stories obtained by SKIGD are presented in this book with cultural analysis and interpretations in relation to their life experiences in Korea and America. They include their emotional state, personality, lifestyle, family and social interactions, religious faith, spirituality, efforts to secure independence, feelings and thoughts about life at an advanced age, illnesses, and death.

Depressives and nondepressives diagnosed with the structured KDIS-III or semistructured SKIGD are interpreted in comparative terms from their own narration, when appropriate.

Telling one's own story is an open, spontaneous, and therapeutic event. Thus, the story becomes a naturally holistic narrative because the person wants to express all the relevant personal stories for healing. Old age is a time for reminiscence, and it helps the elderly to become better historians, to resolve their conflicts, and to make their lives more meaningful.

The dominant collective message from the elderly Korean immigrants through their stories is about overcoming hardships, reconciling conflicts, especially with children, and spiritual transcendence through endurance.

The Korean elders reiterated many times and in many different ways how precious their children were. They live near their children, for their children, and through their children. Korean elders are either in rapture and ecstasy or in sorrow in relation to their children. For this reason, they do their best for their children and they hurt most when their children disappoint them. They are happy when their children distinguish themselves and when they understand and support their parents.

Some of their expressions of unhappiness are: "When my daughter does not want me to live with her, it hurts me more than the pains I felt at my husband's death," or "I bury my dead child in my bosom although I bury others in the ground." Therefore, Korean elders like to tell happy and sad stories woven together with their children's lives. Despite bickering and hard feelings caused by differences in values and conditions, most of the relationships between parents and children seem to be mended in the end. The maintenance of these relationships is considered fundamental and essential to their core ethics, duty, responsibility, morality, harmony, vital energy, and life itself. Harmony in interpersonal relationships is the source of vitality for health and a meaningful life. Parents make conscious efforts toward enhancing harmonious relationships with their children.

The filial duty of children in traditional Korean culture is an unconditional, genuine obligation to their parents to help preserve their health, well-being, and happiness. However, according to the observations made by some of the informants, some children's devotion seems to be conditional and relative depending on the parents' degree of sacrifice and on parental duties and responsibilities. Some informants had difficulty accepting nontraditional gender roles. Nontraditional distribution of labor is practiced in Korean immigrant families. Adult sons are asked by their wives to do housework. This phenomenon makes elderly Koreans angry and sad.

The Korean informants first told of their experiences of anger, sadness, and depression and then related the origin of their physical illnesses to their hardships and stressful life events in Korea and America. Some of the informants complained of Korean popular illnesses. Some informants said they suffered from one or more Korean illnesses and/or symptoms of depression.

Hwabyung or other Korean illness idioms can be considered in the Korean context as a communication medium that can eliminate interpersonal and psychosocial barriers. The individual with *hwabyung* needs an audience to listen, to understand, to agree or to disagree with, and even to confront, console, and heal. *Hwabyung* is used to publicize painful inner conflicts without taking interpersonal risks. The indigenous illness idioms are sanctioned in Korea and in other Korean communities. The purpose of suffering *hwabyung* is to gain understanding, empathy, and sympathy from others who share similar indigenous beliefs and values. People who complain of *hwabyung* may not have any particular mental or physical health problems. They may have anger, frustration, shame, guilt, and overall stress from being lonely, misunderstood, and disrespected, or they may have low self-esteem based on ordinary and extraordinary life events. Some of the informants just complain about these symptoms without mentioning *hwabyung*. These people would like to defend themselves from being misunderstood, from harsh treatment, or from their own inadequacies. Thus, they may express their painful inner feelings and thoughts with bodily sounds and connoted utterances—for example, "the blood dries up"—although most of the time they may not have physical injuries. They feel that they are about to have physical embarrassment with anger, agony, and frustration. In the immature or less cultivated stage, more somatic complaints are expressed than in the mature and highly cultivated life stage of a person. It seems that more cultivated persons may develop fewer ailments. Some, particularly those with a severe condition, may have both objective signs and subjective symptoms, while some may have only subjective symptoms. Examples of such symptoms are:

1. A person complains of a somatic symptom, but may not have the bodily symptom, only a psychosocial frustration.
2. A person complains of a somatic symptom and actually has the physical symptom as well as the related psychosocial frustration.
3. A person complains of a Korean illness such as *hwabyung*, *han*, or *shingyungshayak* but actually does not have any of them or any symptoms, but only psychosocial frustration, such as anger.
4. A person has *hwabyung*, *han*, or *shingyungshayak* and its bodily symptoms, and complains of it and its symptoms as well as psychosocial frustration, such as anger.

Abstract, real, or urgent physical somatic expressions—for instance, in *hwabyung*, anger or depression—are used to express emotional distress. Elderly Koreans appear to psychologize and express their feelings with bodily idioms. But the underlying dynamic is holistic: psychological, physical, social (collective, inter-, and intrapersonal), environmental, cosmological, natural, spiritual, and religious. It includes all internal and external influences. They seem to take the position that verbalization of feelings cannot express and communicate distressing life experiences as effectively as pathophysiological forms of expression. They describe dramatically and rhetorically how they feel and how they hurt in bodily terms. Emotional terms such as distress, anger, frustration, loneliness, or mortification are not strong, clear, or specific enough to let other people know how they feel and from what they suffer. Their expressions may sound exaggerated or unreal. But they are what the Koreans feel, suffer from, and perceive. Some examples: "The blood dries up!"; "The organs and intestines are burning!" (I am worrying restlessly); "The organs and intestines are injured or rotten!" (My mind is hurting); "The organs and intestines are being twisted!" (in extreme anger and stressed condition); or "The organs and intestines are swollen up!" (someone is greedy enough to hurt others). Most of the above expressions are used in perceived agony, mental shock, and situations of extreme helplessness and powerlessness.

Ideally, it is believed that emotional distress should be "digested in the body," that is, resolved by the individual, and should not be ventilated verbally in psychological, somatic, or especially emotional terms, unless the hurtful feelings and thoughts are sanctioned and accepted by others in Korean illness idioms such as *hwabyung*. When hurt feelings are not properly digested, verbal expressions are uttered as in the examples in the previous paragraph. Some people cannot digest them at all due a to lack of self-cultivation or due to a firelike personality.

Elderly Korean immigrants seem to accept almost any diagnosis without any particular preferences or criticisms as long as they are able to communicate their problems, regrets, resentments, distress, anger, anxiety, and so on. Some of the informants used the terms depression and *hwabyung* interchangeably. Some used *hwabyung*, depression, *han,* and *shingyungshayak*. Few people were able to distinguish them. A key informant commented that even older Koreans do not seem to use *hwabyung* exclusively. In a sense, it really does not matter what idioms or diagnoses they use as long as they can communicate and make others understand and they are accepted with sympathy and empathy, not rejected and ostracized by family members, relatives, friends, and neighbors. When such goals are reached, individuals live more peacefully as a result of such self-care and therapy through communication. They are willing to talk about themselves when they know they have a safe communication channel or confidant. Such safe communication is free of retaliation or damage to interpersonal relationships with significant family members such as a son, daughter-in-law, daughter, or grandchildren. This could be called interpersonal healing. Self-care is also expressed physically by taking nature walks or mentally by listening to music for self-cultivation. All these create and promote holistic self-care.

Holistic symptom expression calls for nature-oriented self-care. Self-healing is used to resolve all worries and conflicts through self-cultivation, self-regulation, and sometimes self-blame, by being more generous, patient, and self-sacrificing through mature self-reflection. Especially, those who are religious, moral, and ethical use self-reproach. They believe that they are wrong although they did not do anything wrong in the worldly sense. This could be the notion of "sinning" in Christianity whereas in Buddhism, "karma" might be the idiom. In this case, self-digestion of the irritants (internal resolution of problems), self-cultivation, and accumulation of virtue are some ways to resolve problems. By overcoming anger, there is a new acceptance of the self, with new energy, optimism, and hope. This is true *ch'enyom*. It is almost all resolved internally without hurting oneself, anyone else, or going to a professional psychotherapist. However, some may use confidants.

Ultimately these elderly Koreans reach the truth of accepting "absurd worldly phenomena" such as struggling, suffering, harmful desires, and misunderstanding through reconciliatory religious and/or spiritual transcending and awakening. It initiates and results in a pure mind and body. It is an act of silent physical and psychological nonviolence. This positive force that transforms "evil" thought to harmonious thought and acceptance is called *ch'enyom*. It is reflected in facial expression, equanimity, inner peace, appearance, language, and deeds. This state of mind is possible and relevant, particularly for Koreans in their reminiscences, and for integrity.

Elderly Koreans live dependently with and in nature. Their language reflects the phenomena: "Heaven [part of the cosmos that has an environment as well as a merciful, righteous, humanistic, and godly spiritual character] will help you"; "Aren't you afraid of heaven?"; "Heaven will punish you!" Heaven as an omnipotent provider and a lord is a powerful disciplinarian and trustworthy comforter both somatically and psychologically. Natural energy is used for harmonious health by means of breathing, conducting oneself in a self-cultivated manner, appreciating music, martial arts, singing, body movements, dancing, calligraphy, meditation with breathing in the lotus position, psychologically and somatically satisfying meals, sleeping, using traditional herbs, self-acupressure, and acupuncture for the whole body-mind. The somatic, intra- and inter-emotional and psychosocial efforts are concerted harmoniously. According to Dr. Jong Woo Kim (1998), a traditional Korean physician, harmony is created for a person who suffers from anger and frustration with pure sadness and without grudges. Harmony prevents bodily injury. In other words, sadness acts as a therapeutic element. There is a balance between positive and negative forces and the five elements of traditional medical principles. That might be why Koreans were able to survive during the Japanese occupation, the Korean War, and acculturation and change in America. During those times, their initial reaction to loss could have been anger and then sorrow. Anger and sorrow harmonized as peace of mind.

Another care method is interpersonal harmonious exchange, *chong,* which can consist of doing thoughtful deeds for others out of sympathy or empathy. The health and illness beliefs and practices of elderly Korean immigrants, based on their epistemology, seem to be related to their indigenous nature orientation, with cosmological, religious, and philosophical foundations. All good deeds such as thinking positively of others and oneself, training the body-mind, and harmonizing interpersonal relationships by promoting another's welfare will lead to harmony experienced as peace of mind and, ultimately, holistic health.

Health is related to everyday life. Here is an example: The daughter of an elderly Korean woman notified her that she would receive a bottle of medication from the daughter's husband that would promote her memory. However, for some reason, the mother did not receive it. But when her daughter advised her over the phone to make sure to take the medication, the mother just said, "I will take it as you like me to." The situation was dealt with peacefully and, even though the mother had not received the medication, she did not mind as long as there was harmony in the family. She was able to accept the failure and give a gift of peace to herself and others. In another gesture of goodwill, the mother bought several copies of books on Buddhist meditation that she then distributed to others.

DISCUSSION AND CONCLUSION

Almost all the elders interviewed came to this country to join their children; virtually all initially lived with their adult children and, over time, moved to their own apartments. Some informants regret the fact that they have not done much for the public beyond their own family care. However, most of them did more than their share in surviving the Japanese occupation, poverty, the Korean

War, maltreatment from their spouses, oppression by in-laws and authorities, taking care of their extended family and neighborhood, etc. Instantly, Korean women had to become breadwinners outside the home without training or resources during poverty-stricken wartime. Some claimed that they were victimized in the male-dominated society. An informant was ashamed of herself for her selfish luxury life and her "own immaturity," being "a spoiled brat," because this does not reflect altruistic and virtuous living, but instead shows a lack of self-cultivation.

Most of the informants had to take care of their four-generation extended families with parents-in-law, children, grandchildren, and sometimes brothers- and sisters-in-law as well as their neighborhood and community, in addition to their business or farm work all year.

Their happiness and sickness depend on their children. When the children are doing well themselves and are kind to their parents, of course, their parents are happy. And when they are not, the parents may have depression or *hwabyung*. No factors influence the informants more than their children. Their children are the most precious cause for their existence; that is why they can be so happy, proud, contented, angry, bitter, betrayed, resentful, or regretful about them. Their children are their possessions, and the parents are integrated with their children, whether it is good or bad for most of them. Compare what Gibran (1989:18) writes about children: "Your children are not your children. They are sons and daughters of Life's longing for itself. They come through you but not from you. And though they are with you, yet they belong not to you. You may give them your love but not your thoughts."

Abstract, real, or physically felt or imagined somatic expressions are used to express emotional distress. Elderly Koreans appear to psychologize, but express it in bodily idioms. But the underlying dynamics of somatic expression are holistic although they seem to be only physical: psychological, physical, social (individual, collective, inter- and intrapersonal), environmental, cosmological, naturalistic, and religious. They include all internal and external stimuli. Elderly Koreans seem to take the position that psychologically expressed complaints cannot properly communicate distressing life experiences as effectively as traditional, idiosyncratic, metamorphic, pathophysiological idioms. They attempt to express how they feel and how they hurt because of psychosocially, morally, and ethically originated and felt insults, indignation, and distress in bodily idioms. For example, "It was as painful as though I was stricken a hundred times by a huge, sharp, and yet heavy saber."

To maintain and promote virtuous and harmonious relationships between children and parents, the informants use certain cognitive, emotional, and behavioral self-help strategies. These strategies include *ch'enyom* (right thinking and behaviors), along with *nunchi* (learning what is going on with people around oneself in order to react accordingly), unconditional sacrifice, *chong* (compassionate behaviors and expressions), and parental duty. Some of the elderly Koreans seem almost to reach sainthood. They are expected to be that way. If they are not free of "immaturity or lack of cultivation," they are discouraged and ridiculed. *Chong* can be considered as caring for others, which also acts as self-help for the caregiver. The disappearance of an existing "lump" of distress by storytelling and sharing may bring relief, especially when it is channeled through the supportive roles of loving, active listeners. Multireligious influences on the healing process are reflected. *Chong* and fate, motivating forces, help Korean elders mobilize to live courageously.

Most of the Korean informants, including the depressives diagnosed with KDIS-III, function as nondepressives in Korea and America. They work at home to raise their children and outside to earn money. They were not hospitalized and they took no medicine. This leads us to feel that people should be diagnosed and treated differently according to the individual's holistic being, actions, and cultural orientation.

PART I: ETHOS, HEALTH, AND ILLNESS

Chapter 1

Theoretical Foundation

THE URGE TO TELL STORIES

Wan-Suh Park, a renowned Korean writer who is also a daughter, daughter-in-law, wife, mother, mother-in-law, and grandmother, described in her short story "In the Realm of Buddha" her emotions, thoughts, and behaviors as she experienced family deaths during the Korean War. She wrote her story to relieve the wound she felt in her soul and body (Park, 1996).

Ferrara (1994) says that the sharing of self in discourse with someone is finding a place in the world, and that is why it is therapeutic. Some people write what is in their minds and souls, perhaps because they cannot find suitable people to listen to their stories, or because they want to share them with as many people as possible.

DEPRESSION

The following review of literature related to depression was done with a focus on elderly Korean immigrants. Coryell and associates (1995:1124) wrote "characteristics of people with untreated major depressive disorder were: old age, the presence of disruption in role function, longer durations, psychosocial impairment, and having serious economic disadvantages." Suicide rates among Koreans, Japanese, and Chinese seemed to increase with age (Kalish, 1968). Fear of unmet dependency needs is a common source of depressive symptoms (Blatt and Zuroff, 1992). The wife who feels that she lacks emotional support may experience depressive symptoms

(Brown and Harris, 1978). Will elderly Korean immigrants exhibit these symptomatic phenomena?

In the Depner and Ingersoll-Dayton (1985) study, emotional support was defined as confiding, reassurance, and talking things over when upset. Nolen-Hoeksema (1987) stated that women adapt to depressive experiences by ruminating, especially about the quality of their close relationships, which makes the symptoms worse, while men respond to depressive experiences by engaging in increased activity. It will be interesting to find out what might be therapeutic for Koreans.

Culture and Depression

Depressive experiences are universal but can be unique according to sociocultural variations. However, there is a relative paucity of basic research on the psychosocial aspects of depression (Kleinman, 1986). Cultural variations exist in origin, expression, and adaptation of depression (Good, Good, and Moradi, 1985; Kleinman, 1986). "Depression is experienced by the sufferer as a reality, a set of symptoms or a condition expressed and interpreted in local idioms and using local explanatory frames. Depression as a condition of the sufferer is interpreted secondarily by family members, caregivers, and others in the society" (Good, Good, and Moradi, 1985: 381). "All symptoms have personal significance and are inherently 'culturally patterned'" (Good and Good, 1981: 177). A symptom or illness contains "a network of meanings for the sufferer: personal trauma, life stresses, fears and expectations about the illness, social reactions of friends and authorities, and therapeutic experiences" (Good and Good, 1981: 176). Even the same disease may show itself through different symptoms in different ethnic groups. Angel and Thoits (1987) stated that cognitive and linguistic categories of illness characteristics of any culture constrain the interpretative and behavioral options available to individuals in response to symptoms.

Kirmayer (1989) stated that excessive emotional expression might interfere with interpersonal relationships and trigger major psychiatric disorders in vulnerable family members. This might apply to Korean elders because they may still hold the necessary cultural values and seemingly somatic but emotional idioms in communicating depression and other negative emotions.

Depression has been defined in broad and divergent terms. Depression is characterized as a feeling, a reaction, a syndrome, and an illness (Silverman, 1968). Kirmayer (1989) concluded that distress is experienced and expressed socioculturally, and the way an illness is labeled may be related to personality, fate, idiom, or sociomoral situations.

Lutz (1985:91) points out that the distinction between cognitive and affective domains is not seen in every culture. Among the Ifaluk of the Pacific, "Emotions may be grouped with moral values rather than (or as much as) with internal disruption. They may be linked with logical thoughts as much as or more than internal conflict, and they may be seen as characteristics of situations or relationships rather than as the property of individuals."

Symptoms vary both intraculturally (Kirmayer, 1989) and cross-culturally (Kleinman, 1980). I expect there are phenomenological differences among individuals. There may be a specific Korean way of dealing with depressive experiences. Local equivalent names for depression, etiology, manifestation, course, treatment regimen, and prevention of depression can be different in non-Western cultural groups and can differ from culture to culture. These differences are largely not known across cultures.

Concepts such as dependency, depression, anxiety, aggression, anger, jealousy, death, love, suicide, and humanity are not the same across cultures (Marsella and Kameoka, 1989). "Feeling blue" and "feeling guilty" are not typical Asian complaints in depression. The Japanese term for depression, *yuutsu*, uses nature metaphors (rain, storm, dark, mountains) (Sakauye et al., 1994). These conditions signal the need for cross-cultural communication to facilitate health promotion and maintenance.

Cheung, Law, and Waldman (1981) examined the symptom presentation of depressed patients seen at a general medical clinic in Hong Kong. According to this study, not all depressed patients were aware of their depressed mood, and most did not complain primarily of their emotional distress. The range of symptoms was not different from those experienced by nondepressed patients with medical disorders. However, depressed patients frequently complained of vague and diffuse somatic symptoms that concealed the depressive mood, but when they were directly questioned about their mood, most of the depressed patients admitted to feelings of sadness. The authors concluded that somatization as a way of manifesting depression may involve different psychological processes. The depressed person may have to somatize to avoid social stigma attributed to mental illness instead of verbalizing dysphoria.

Depression and Somatization

Somatization has been defined by Katon, Kleinman, and Rosen (1982) as both the expression of physical complaints in the absence of defined organic pathology and the amplification of symptoms resulting in a psychiatric condition influencing the number of somatization symptoms (Escobar et al., 1987). Depression is commonly associated with somatization (Kleinman, 1982). Also, somatization has been reported in the absence of psychopathology as an expression of and means of interpreting and coping with personal distress and social stress (Katon, Kleinman, and Rosen, 1982; Kleinman, 1980). Somatization is the common way of expressing distress among Koreans (Kim and Rhi, 1976: 107; Baik, 1984: 291).

In Korean traditional medicine there is a certain set of symbolic functions for each body organ. For example, the lungs are related to worrying, sorrow, and low spirit, and depression means malfunction of the liver and the kidneys (Kim and Rhi, 1976: 104).

Kang (1981), a professional Korean traditional physician and professor, stated that diseases have internal causes. For example, there are seven emotions: happiness, anger, depression, brooding, sorrow, fear, and startling. These emotions are related to mental function. If mental stimulation is too severe, the emotions become excessive, and this state could trigger diseases in major vital body organs, due to the relationship of mind, emotion, and body. S. H. Lee (1977) pointed out that emotional and mental agony brings along physical problems and pain, which he calls psychogenic pain. He explained that an individual would have amplified bodily pains when depressed.

Kleinman states that somatization may be regarded as "a particular cognitive-behavioral type whose adaptive or maladaptive consequences would involve assessment of particular social and cultural as much as personal variables" (Kleinman, 1982: 130). Later, Kleinman (1995: 9) states: "Somatization seems normative and often normal; it is not so much a substitution for something but a more basic way of being-in-the-world. . . . Somatic modes of experience now seem to me better understood in a sociosomatic language." Kleinman (1995: 10-11) interpreted somatization as "an idiom of interpersonal distress, a form of cultural experience rooted as much in political and social structural processes as in clinical ones. Depression, too, I recast as a relationship between person and society."

Depression is not sanctioned in China, but somatization is sanctioned because depression is considered a stigmatized mental illness (Kleinman and Kleinman, 1985: 478).

Depression and Popular Illnesses Among Koreans

Few depressive patients seem to be diagnosed among Koreans (Hahn, 1965; Kim and Rhi, 1976). In Korean culture, depression is not clearly understood. Depression is likely to be expressed as *hwabyung* (physical-emotional distress), *shingyungshayak* (psychologically and neurotically based physical syndromes), or *han* (passive expression of regrets and resentment). These are Korean popular illnesses. In a study about the cultural construction of illness, one person out of the sample of twenty elderly Korean immigrant women suffered from depression, and all others related their bodily symptoms to *hwabyung* (Pang, 1991). S. H. Lee (1977) stated that *hwabyung* is an anger syndrome.

Lin (1983) studied *hwabyung*. His patients were preoccupied more with somatic symptoms than behavioral or psychological symptoms. Their examples of somatic complaints were indigestion, anorexia, dysphoria, palpitations, generalized pains and aches, and epigastric masses, which were not confirmed on physical examination. Some of the other complaints were insomnia, fatigue, morbid fear of impending death, and dysphoria. The patients responded well to antidepressants and supportive therapy. Lin recommended that *hwabyung* should be studied further as a culture-bound syndrome and depression "as a relatively cultural-free psychiatric diagnostic category" (1983: 106-107).

Han seems to represent dysphoric affects such as self-pity, depression, and sadness that are associated commonly with frustrations, hostility, and grudges because of disappointments in life and unfulfilled dreams, hopes, and aspirations. *Han* may be caused by the self in its attitude toward others or by others through means of oppression, disloyalty, unfaithfulness, negligence, and deprivation of happiness and well-being. The common regrets about the negligent care of parents or children seem to be called guilt by Westerners and shame or *han* in Korea. *Han* includes many other meanings. Guilt feelings were expressed by Korean patients twice as often as by Indian patients. The guilt of the Korean depressives had a social and family orientation, without religious overtones (Kim, K., 1997).

Kleinman (1982) states that the Chinese complain of neurasthenia when they have depressionlike symptoms. In Korea, too, neurasthenia seems to be a familiar name for depressionlike physical and psychological symptoms.

KOREAN ETHOS

Some Korean emotions, thoughts, and behaviors that operate in everyday life will be discussed in this section. Self-concept in Korea is related to the ego's various interpersonal and group relationships, such as family, friends, country, etc. Furthermore, self-concept among Koreans includes ancestors, nature, and the cosmos in relation to natural and supernatural power based on Korean and Far East Asian philosophical and religious backgrounds. Thus, Baik (1984: 283-286) termed the self-concept of Koreans as "all inclusive self." This self-concept orientation tends to foster obedience, self-sacrifice for group goals, and group harmony. Yielding and sacrificing for others, rather than self-realization, are considered primary virtues. Therefore, individual-centered self-fulfilling actions in the Western sense may be somewhat different among Koreans. S. H. Lee (1987) notes that Koreans tend not to say what they really think, in order not to offend or confront others. This is considered a virtue (Rhi, 1986). The self is masked in the interest of finding harmony and adjustment with others and with the environment.

Chong is said to be a unique warm emotion between or among people, and it promotes caring behaviors toward those to whom one feels close. *Chong* might be something like true humanistic, loving, caring, and thoughtful behaviors. It can occur among all people and in all relationships. Erotic love may or may not contain *chong*. *Chong* can be expressed to anyone and can be received from anyone. Erotic love is usually limited to one or a few people. *Chong* could be seen as erotic, agape, or the two combined. According to L. Kim (1991), *chong* promotes the depth and richness of the relationship. It brings people together and encourages empathic and sympathetic feelings. *Chong* closes the gap of emotional isolation. In times of social unrest or personal crisis, *chong* supports and sustains caring, gentle, loyal, constant, considerate, devoted, sacrificial, and nurturing human relationships. It is a subtle, caring love, as opposed to erotic love. It can exist in various relationships, such as between a child and parents, between husband and wife, between student and teacher, among friends, between employee and employer, between customer and businessperson, etc. The nature, quality, or degree of *chong* is different according to the kinds of relationship that people have.

MIND-BODY-NATURE CULTIVATION IN KOREA

Koreans believe that where the will is, there is energy; where energy is, there is blood; where blood is, there is vitality. The center of the cosmos is the mind, which creates the body. The energy of the cosmos is our energy. The will of the cosmos is our will. Physical health and peace of mind are the roots of a high standard of self-cultivation. The cultivated person is free from anger and extreme frustration.

Religion, education, philosophy, economics, sociology, medicine, arts, and sports all come from one root. The real image of life should be understood to realize the full functioning of harmonious human-nature relationships (Lee, 1990). The mind initiates and influences how one thinks and behaves and what one creates.

Asian culture emphasizes harmony with people and the environment instead of antagonism or mastery. To preserve harmony with people, indirect communication is often used. Silence is sometimes used to communicate disagreement nonverbally. Confrontation may be viewed as aggressive, causing conflict and making the situation worse because harmony is disturbed (Chin, 1993).

ANCESTORS, FAMILY, AND FILIAL PIETY IN KOREA

All sons are expected to have the responsibility and obligation for their aged parents' well-being because of the reciprocal dependence of successive generations. Parents may depend on all their sons because all their sons have depended on them. Each son has a debt from his early years that has to be repaid. Yet the offspring can never repay their parents fully for the gift of life, for the affection, luxury, and sacrifices that parents so freely bestow and grant. A common Korean example of filial piety, as found in famous folk stories, is the feeding of one's own flesh and blood to aged and ill parents as nutrients and medicine for recovery. When the study of Confucianism was instituted in Korea during the seventh and eighth centuries A.D., the *Hyo Kyong* (a Chinese classic on filial piety) was the first text adopted (Yi, 1973: 8). In the late nineteenth century, C. Dallet, a French missionary, observed: "No virtue in Korea is esteemed and honored as much as filial piety, none is taught with more care, none is more magnificently recompensed by exemptions from taxes, by the erection of monumental columns or even temples, and by honors and public offices" (Dallet, 1954: 137).

The important beliefs and expected practices of filial piety are submission, attendance, support, comfort of parents, realization of parents' wishes, the provision of funeral services, and ancestor worship (Choi, 1964; Janelli and Janelli, 1982). The children and grandchildren who venerate their Korean elders will become leaders for the ancestor worship ceremony in appreciation of their elders' sufferings for their children. It is considered most shameful, pitiful, and even sinful if children fail to fulfill their filial piety to their elderly parents.

A folk story called "Koryojang" recounts unfilial behavior. The parents in a poor family are elderly, infirm, and their children think they are useless. They are taken far away to a mountain where there is nothing to eat and no place to sleep, and left all alone. A slightly different version of the story says that an elder is left in a hut with some food. He or she may starve to death or be eaten by wild animals or buried alive in a mud pot.

The two extremes, the filial and the unfilial, have been compared in this discussion. Also, all my life I have heard the expression, "There is no filial son for a long illness." However, Koreans have a stronger belief in filial piety than "Koryojang" shows. Certainly, there are challenging tasks in caring for Korean elders in relation to one's duty, responsibility, reality, and morality.

Traditionally, marriage is negotiated between two parties based on socially recognized norms. A woman's opinion does not count in her own marriage decision. Her father and her future husband's father traditionally make the decision. The woman belongs to three men in her life. Before marriage a woman is to obey her father; after marriage, her husband; and in old age, her son. Her marriage is not always secure. A woman can be sent back to her parents' home if she shows any of the following seven "evils": disobedience to parents-in-law, adultery, jealousy, barrenness, an incurable disease, a quarrelsome disposition, or theft (Lee, 1967:137). In such cases she would suffer from stigma throughout her life and she would bring shame to her husband's home, her parents' home, and herself (Pang, 1991). The obedience to parents, particularly to parents-in-law, is emphasized most strongly.

After marriage, any conflicts between the bride and other members of the family would be expected to be resolved in the in-laws' favor (Harvey, 1979). According to a popular saying, Korean women who enter marriage are frequently advised to become dumb for the first three years, deaf another three years, and blind for three years after that to survive, particularly in the early phase of marriage. Blind obedience is expected and is considered a virtue.

Obedience, suppression of wishes, and nonreciprocal conformity are expected principles of socialization in Korean women (Harvey, 1979). This quality or virtue is the foundation for filial piety and harmony in a household. Filial piety is the sine qua non or basic quality for a decent family member or citizen with integrity, esteem, and dignity. Filial piety is the standard criterion for a cultivated man or woman.

A newly married daughter-in-law works under the constant supervision of her mother-in-law, from whom she is expected to learn the family customs and traditions. A bride should respect and obey her mother-in-law. However, there are many examples of conflicts. Consequently, nowadays some mothers-in-law move out of their son's household and some daughters-in-law commit suicide.

PROVERBS REFLECTING KOREAN VALUES

Proverbs are the foundation for understanding a people's culture, ethos, and values (Chung, 1995; Ha, 1964). Some proverbs demonstrate hope and optimism among Koreans: "Even if the sky falls down, there is a hole or a way to survive," or "Even if you happen to be caught in a tiger's den, if only you are alert and do your best, you will survive." Some proverbs symbolize natural and spiritual providence: "If you have been starving for three days, surely there will be someone who would bring you something to eat," or "The wind blows and blows and then it finally stops."

As the Korean proverb states: "The mouth is the executioner and the doctor of the body." According to Chung (1995), this saying is related to the importance of nutrition. However, to the author, it is also related to verbalization. Kind and gentle words could be healing and "sharp tongues" could literally kill people.

Some adages sound passive but have very powerful humanistic, peacemaking, and disciplinary messages: "Losing is winning." "Winning is losing." "If one is patient for an hour, he or she will be peaceful for one hundred days" and "If there were only three letters *[yin nae sim]* meaning patience, even killing would be prevented." Koreans are taught these kinds of values through proverbs.

Koreans like to think and talk about fate. In a similar vein, misfortune, illness, and disease are understood in terms of karma and fate. One has to suffer and endure heavy burdens in life, but there are ways to overcome them. Their hardships can be lightened or can disappear depending on one's mental attitude. Tribulation can be regarded rationally. Agonizing experience is ultimately survived by the individual (Shin, 1983).

"A deaf person who suffers from chest illness," refers to a person who lives in oppressed, insecure conditions with feelings of inferiority or vulnerability, where there is no freedom or right to speak what one feels, knows, desires, or dislikes, and no freedom to act as one chooses.

Other proverbs are related to the parental care of children. "Although a parent can take care of ten children, ten children cannot take care of a parent" and "There is Buddha inside a parent, but there is obstinacy inside a child." "There is love downward [to children], but there is no love upward [to parents]." In other words, there is love from parents to children but sometimes there is little love from children to parents. Parents are parental but children are unfilial. Essentially, the proverbs mean that parents are to love and care and children are to be loved and cared for. Still, parents can influence their children. "Good sons are born to good parents." It may be related to "Love goes where love comes."

The proverbs relating to the sorrows of widows are: "A young widow's wailing makes mountains, sky, grass, and trees—the whole world—cry." "The sound of a young widow's crying makes heaven cry." "As a young widow sighs, the frost will come all over." "A widow understands a widow's heart, mind, and soul." These adages show that a widow's sorrows cannot be exaggerated.

Proverbs also reflect opinions and feelings about daughters-in-law: "If the daughter-in-law is considered mean, so is the grandson," "The daughter-in-law brings disgrace to the family," or "If a family is to be ruined, a daughter-in-law will grow whiskers." A daughter-in-law said to have whiskers may mean that she has become unyielding and dauntless enough to be authoritative and masculine, when a typical daughter-in-law should behave in a most feminine and obedient way. It may refer to a situation where a daughter-in-law takes over or controls the whole household and threatens the traditional family patriarchal, hierarchical order originating from Confucianism. It is expressed very well in another proverb: "If a hen crows, the family will be in ruin." An ideal daughter-in-law is expected to obey her parents-in-law by knowing her role, the expectations of others, and by staying in their household until she dies no matter how difficult conditions are in the extended family.

Also, there are some sayings about old age and death: "Death itself is not sad but growing old is a pity," "Dying is not sad but having aches and pains is sorrowful," "To die suddenly is best," etc.

These proverbs convey the desire for a full and wholesome life to the end. And dying and death should not be too bad after all.

SELF-CARE

Self-care may have therapeutic efficacy. Self-care with meditation based on nature and religion appears to be very important among elderly Koreans. In the Korean cultural context, it is very natural for old people, whether sick or well, to turn to nature's healing power to refresh the body and mind through meditation, spending time quietly in the mountains surrounded by trees or by the sea in clean air. Koreans may also be familiar and comfortable in the atmosphere of shamanism, Buddhism, Confucianism, and other religions. The synthesis of multiple religions seems to empower elderly Korean immigrants to be confident enough to take care of themselves. It may be true that Koreans feel a sense of belonging and protection even in the absence of tangible support because of their inner spiritual strength founded on multiple religions.

The conflicts and frustrations of changing immigrant life seem to be solved when they relinquish their needs and wishes and accept their situations without demanding anything. The reasons some people employ a self-care approach and some do not differ. Koreans may employ *ch'enyom*, a Buddhist concept of mental discipline. It can aid in regaining emotional balance, renewing spiritual, religious, and holistic power, and composing themselves, family, and others. They find inner peace with themselves and others. In Korea, "giving up" or *ch'enyom* is more synonymous with "resigning oneself" or "yielding" to others than with "abandoning hope." It involves relinquishing one's desires toward and expectations of others and accepting one's *p'alcha*, or destiny, in harmony with the cosmos. The term *ch'enyom* actually has a meaning much more profound than that in common usage. *Ch'e* means truth, self-awareness, and clarification in Buddhist terms. *Ch'enyom* is the ancient translation of *chongsa,* right thinking, the second component of the Buddhist Eightfold Path (Rhi, 1986; 252-253). Buddhism emphasizes the teaching, "Since I have no self that is separate and isolated from you, therefore I must care for you" (Park, 1995). In other words, all people should help one another to be harmonious and wholesome together. Mutual nurturing is indispensable for self, for others, and for the whole universe.

Koenig, George, and Siegler (1988) found that among older adults accepting their situation is a coping mechanism. To the elderly, accepting means having done the best they could, and still doing the best they can in the situation. Having done everything they could to solve problems, they accept them and get on with their lives. Acceptance enables an individual to divert attention from stressors to more meaningful activities. Acceptance is effective only when all possible attempts have been made to resolve problems and the situation is no longer under the direct control of the individual.

Murphy (1982) remarked that the majority of older persons who are suffering from social problems, adverse life events, and poor health remain remarkably cheerful; it is only those who lack a confidant who appear to be vulnerable to depression in the face of these problems. Murphy considered that a confidant could act as a buffer. She went on to propose that an essential protective quality is the capacity for intimacy. This, it should be emphasized, it is an attribute not of the confidant but of the individual's own personality.

Ki-baik Lee's book titled *A New History of Korea* (1984) was dedicated to the people of Korea: "That the record of those enduring qualities of strength, and fortitude, and cultural creativity that so distinguish their long, proud history may become more widely known" (p. 4). Self-sufficiency and self-confidence among Koreans are byproducts of their endurance of hardships and various historical forms of oppression, such as Japanese colonialism (Eckert et al., 1990). Yun (1976) stated that endurance has been an essential psychological quality for the survival of individual Koreans, as well as for the nation: a kind of moderation that refers to a restrained, sparing, and temperate state of mind. It seems to reflect Koreans' strong self-sufficiency in every aspect of life, including nature- and nurture-oriented health and self-care.

Weil (1995) points out the body's innate natural power to heal itself. Gordon (1996) describes the healing process in changing one's attitude about life and interpersonal relationships in addition to natural multicultural healing methods. Kuo and Tsai (1986) hypothesize that immigrants are not only reactive to stressful life changes. Rather, the chief means of ameliorating strain is the immigrant's activism in cultivating social networks and strength of personality. Park (1990) talks about the need for cognitive turning around. For example, one can believe, "Yes, my god will spare me." Those who can do that will be able to console themselves. The help of others goes only so far. The individual is responsible for the rest (Sim, 1995). Ultimately, various ways of supernatural and spiritual caring are sought. Projections toward supernatural beings are another common way of coping with distress (Baik, 1984; Kim and Rhi, 1976; S. H. Lee, 1977).

Confucians believe that health and illness are controlled by divine fate in heaven. According to Taoism, men who conduct their lives in accordance with the doctrine of Tao accumulate essence that allows their spirits to realize their full potential and preserve harmony (Unschuld, 1985). In Korea, 80 percent of the population has some affiliation to a religion. Prominent religions include Christianity, Buddhism, Confucianism, Taoism, and shamanism (K. I. Kim et al., 1993; Chung, 1995; S. B. Park, 1995). One of the Buddha's fundamental insights is the recognition that everybody suffers from illness, growing old, death, separation from loved ones, and unfulfilled desires. It is said to be possible to end this pain by following "the Eightfold Way—correct views, correct intentions, correct speech, correct behaviors, correct living, correct effort, correct attitude, and correct concentration" (Unschuld, 1985:135). According to the Buddha, every action is evil if it harms others and/or one's self (Unschuld, 1985). Korean Confucianism emphasizes emotional control in order to cultivate harmonious hierarchical interpersonal relationships, especially with elders (Rhi, 1986).

Koreans with shamanistic inclinations may enjoy experiencing the ecstasy of spirit possession, but often they are not prepared to face the postecstatic state (Rhi, 1980; Kim, K. I., 1991). Shamans in Korea may experience extreme emotions differently from Buddhists or Confucians. Confucians are known for suppressing emotions (Rhi, 1983), being intellectual, and not being superstitious. In this environment, affinity or closeness to natural and supernatural forces is encouraged and fostered.

Taoism, Buddhism, Confucianism, and shamanism are important cultural inheritances that have had great influence on the Korean personality (Kim and Rhi, 1976). There are strong psychotherapeutic elements in Taoism, such as the process and method of developing insight into one's mind. Taoism alleviates the existential anxiety of the average person, as well as pathological anxiety (Kim and Rhi, 1976). Principles of the Tao point out that the self can direct the self or others toward therapeutic efficacy. Following the principles of Tao is a wise, pure, understanding, forgiving, open, deep, vast, dignified, and visionary way of living.

According to K. T. Lee (1992), among Koreans emotions such as happiness and sorrow spring up and flow from the stomach. Koreans say that when they are glad, the umbilicus laughs. Goodness is expressed as "white belly" and evil as "dark belly." Determination, wisdom, thought, and even chastity are understood in terms of the stomach. The stomach can hold also all sorts of distress, regrets, betrayal, shame, guilt, rage, and agony. To get rid of these, Koreans sing *tchang,* with thirty-six various voice styles that can be expressed as winding, pushing, stamping, knitting, cutting, sprinkling, pressing, etc. with strenuous emotional and skillful physical efforts. Another way of removing distress or *hwabyung* is by stamping on dried gourd bowls and breaking them. Remedies such as these have been used as powerfully efficacious indigenous ways of healing, in harmony with their cultural context, although they may not be widely recognized by Koreans. Korean traditional dance is also used to get rid of conflicts, distress, or ills. T. K. Lee (1987) pointed out that the gestures and movements of Korean folk dancing are symbols for removing worries, distresses, conflicts, etc. Thus, in Korea, arts such as music and dance are used to express and resolve distress.

OTHER REMEDIES

Morita therapy (to accept reality; e.g., the weakness of self) and *Naikan* therapy (to transform feelings of bitterness stemming from mistreatment into gratitude toward others by acknowledging what one received from others) do not require psychological explanations among the Japanese (Ohnuki-Tierney, 1984). These approaches may have influenced the Korean self-healing process through multiple religious and spiritual roots.

Reminiscing has therapeutic efficacy in individuals and groups. It is growth oriented and enables people to find commonalities with one another. The elderly place themselves in a life-span perspective and compare their lives to those of others. They also gain a more supportive foundation in the past and present (Burnside, 1994). Cook (1988) indicated that the theme of war in her research elicited sad memories; however, such sharing could have been a catharsis. Reminiscences can alleviate depression. They can cause improvement in self-regard and lead to current problem solving and existential self-understanding (Burnside, 1994).

The use of reminiscing therapy can give the participants a sense of identity and have positive effects on their social interactions. It also allows for the resolution of previous conflicts and worries, which could be very useful for participants who are caught up in traditional ways of expressing their depression. Music is used to help evoke memories and encourage members to share their thoughts (Burnside, 1994).

K. T. Lee (1977) made the observation that Koreans try to resolve conflicts and emotional distress, induced by others or by themselves, internally and indirectly. Westerners try to deal externally with their emotional or mental concerns or with their problems with other people. Koreans may carry grudges inside and become depressed by them, while Westerners may not harbor grudges so often. Koreans who are immature in their self-resolution process may hurt or torture themselves to take revenge, or they may hurt a victor indirectly by inducing guilt or bringing shame on the person.

K. T. Lee (1987) stated that human emotion is formless, colorless, tasteless, invisible, and intangible. However, when emotional feelings are oppressed, a physical lump is formed, usually in the stomach or throat, that hardens and becomes knotted. The process of lumping is called *han,* regret and resentment or agony; the process of knotting is called *won*, grudge, spite, or grievance.

Ae Jin Hong, who was taken to China to serve as a comfort woman during the Japanese occupation, said the lumps in her chest were resolved after she had an opportunity to tell about her cruel experience to an interviewer from Korea, her motherland (Comfort Women Research Committee, 1995).

Korean history is a history of oppression. Koreans have been oppressed nationally by politicians, rulers, the rich, and the aristocrats. Morally, three bonds have oppressed them: strict rules in the relationships of king and subject; father and son; and husband and wife. They have also been restrained and disciplined by five moral rules that govern human relations: of king and subject with righteousness and loyalty; of father and son with compassion and respect; husband and wife with discretion and distance; brothers observing seniority; and friends trusting each other. All of these are related to Confucian teaching. In addition, there are patriarchal family rules and filial obligations: descendants to ancestors; wife to husband; children to adults; and daughter-in-law to mother-in-law.

Lumps and knots can be painful, and they may interfere with physical functions such as digestion or breathing. There seem to be subtle distinctions between *han* and *won,* although K. T. Lee (1987) does not distinguish specifically. *Han* is brooding within the self about actions one regrets, mainly one's own actions, and about the cruel actions of others. *Won* is active hatred toward others, and it can include plans for revenge.

Korean traditional medicine has been influenced by Chinese traditional medical practices, in which the biological and psychological aspects of illness are interrelated. These practices have been brought into the Korean medical system with specific principles and medicines. "It was known that the various emotions that had been defined were directly anchored in the biological organism and could also influence it. Excessive anger, it was recognized, eventually led to liver damage; fear strained the kidneys. Conversely, this biological integration of emotions also meant that what initially is a purely somatic effect, such as that produced by the influence of cold or excessive physical exertion, can also cause psychic disorders" (Unschuld, 1985: 216). The interrelation between emotion and somatic integrity is evident: excessive emotion will affect bodily integrity and vice versa. Those who experience extreme emotional distress may feel that their somatic integrity is endangered and may say things such as, "My blood will dry up." This might be expressed in a state of near panic to warn others when one is in a terrible situation. This lets others know that it is no longer just an emotional situation but that one is about to lose physical, structural, and functional integrity. It could still be considered a somatization, but it might be seen as a new way of interpretation and a new systematic way of looking at emotion and bodily relationships.

KOREAN IMMIGRANTS AND DEPRESSION

An epidemiological study of depression (Kuo, 1984) stated that Korean immigrants showed the highest prevalence of depression among Asian Americans. Among Chinese, Filipinos, Japanese, and Koreans, the Koreans have the highest mean score, 14.37 on the Center for Epidemiological Studies Depression Scale, followed by Filipinos at 9.72, the Japanese at 7.30, and the Chinese at 6.93. The newer immigrants, exemplified by the Koreans, are more likely to experience excessive adjustment problems in their new society. According to 1990 census data, there are 798,849 Korean residents in the United States, and the population size increased 125 percent since the 1980 census (U.S. Bureau of the Census, 1990).

The American experience of the Korean immigrant has been described in a continuum of euphoria and dysphoria in Korean popular literature (Epstein, 1995). Elderly Korean immigrants' dependency on their children has begun to be reduced, although it has been the children's duty to support their aged parents and let them live in their own home for an indefinite time (B. Kim, 1980: 153-154). This factor and other sociocultural and economic problems may be related to significant depressive experiences as a provoking agent (Brown and Harris, 1978) or to the social origin of depression (Kleinman, 1986; Kleinman and Good, 1985).

Chapter 2

Method

The search for meaning and interpretation of depression and sadness among elderly Korean immigrants is the focus of this book. In the United States, the Diagnostic Interview Schedule (DIS-III) is a screening tool used by professionals as well as laypersons to diagnose mental disorders, including depression. The questions reflect the DSM-III (American Psychiatric Association, 1980) criteria for major depression. In seeking to develop a survey instrument, the Korean Diagnostic Interview Schedule (KDIS), to measure major depression, Lee and associates (Lee et al., 1986) identified a drawback in the DIS-III. The instrument includes a "mood question" that asks informants whether they have felt depressed. Most Koreans—even those suffering from some of the major symptoms of depression—would not admit to being depressed. Cross-cultural modifications to the instrument were made by asking an additional question. The informants are asked the DIS-III question about mood; then the interviewer repeats the question, asking the informant to confirm his or her response. This gives the informant an opportunity to reconsider the answer "no." Since Korean culture discourages informants from admitting to depression, the repeated question, with or without dysphoric mood, allows the interviewer to capture cases of depression. Lee et al. (1986) also added Korean culture-related symptoms to KDIS.

Our work is based on the life stories of elderly Korean immigrants. The stories were obtained by using the Semistructured Korean Interview Guide for Depression (SKIGD), which was designed for Korean immigrants. In consultation with a medical anthropologist, a sociologist, and a historian, the author developed this tool and pilot-tested it. The SKIGD asks a series of questions related to adaptation to old age, adaptation to immigration, experiences of sadness and depression, and experiences of Korean illnesses.

The SKIGD takes approximately three hours to administer in Korean and invites the informant to establish a genuine conversation with the interviewer, touching on the past (e.g., "What hardships and suffering have you had in your life?"), the present, health problems, family, and friends.

SAMPLE

According to 1990 census data, there are 798,849 Korean residents in the United States. Approximately 33 percent reside in California, 12 percent in New York, and 5 percent in Illinois (U.S. Bureau of the Census, 1990). The KDIS was administered to 674 elderly Korean immigrants living in the Washington, DC, metropolitan area. The development of a list of possible interviewees began with the telephone directory and was updated annually. Families from the directory were supplemented by additional names of elderly immigrants gathered from individual and family contacts, churches, and organizations for elderly Koreans. This process yielded a population of 995 individuals who met the criteria of being over age sixty, born in Korea, and now living in the United States. Using an iterative process of selecting every fifth person, a sample of 230 subjects was then decided upon to interview by KDIS to identify informants with major depression. Some of the potential subjects' reasons for not participating included fear of giving information that they should not reveal, being too busy, and being too tired. In a few instances, potential interviewees said their children would not permit them to be interviewed. These 230 subjects, in turn, introduced other potential subjects from their networks, adding 444 additional informants to the sample, for a total of 674 informants. Although network sampling (Sirkin, 1970) reduces the screening cost, it introduces a possible snowballing effect. To avoid having a few informants dominate the selection of the sample, each informant was permitted to name up to three acquaintances.

Two subsamples were drawn: a sample of thirty-four cases who were diagnosed with major depression, and a random sample of thirty-five others who were diagnosed as without major depression. These two subsamples were interviewed with SKIGD in Korean by interviewers who were familiar with Korean culture. Two- to three-hour SKIGD interviews were done, usually at each informant's home. The interviewers had a background of working with elderly Koreans and were familiar with Korean culture. One of the interviewers had mental health training and experience. Tape recordings were made. Interview guides were filled out during each interview with important notes, and later the tape was transcribed into Korean. The informants signed consent forms for participation in the research. The interviews took place from June 1991 to August 1992. I translated the transcribed interview data from Korean into English in consultation with a Koreanist, key informants, and cross-cultural Korean-English and English-Korean references.

MEANING AND INTERPRETATION OF "STORIES ABOUT EVERYDAY LIFE"

Telling one's life story is similar to writing an autobiography. Coles and Coles (1978: v) state, " . . . fine biographies give us both a glimpse of ourselves and a reflection of the human spirit. Biography illuminates history, inspires by example and fires the imagination to life's possibilities. Good biography can create for us lifelong models. Reading about the experiences of others encourages us to persist, to face hardship, and to feel less alone. Biography tells us about choice, steadfastness, and chance."

Storytelling is one of the most significant human behaviors. The act of a person telling about an event to someone else (Smith, 1980) serves many social and cultural purposes but may be viewed primarily as a way of relating individual experience to larger explanatory sociocultural contexts (Brody, 1987). Thus, stories represent an important mode by which people organize, display, and work through experiences. Gee states, "Probably the primary way human beings make sense of their experience is by casting it in narrative form" (1985: 11). Cohler writes that personal narratives are "the most internally consistent interpretation of the presently understood past, experience present, and anticipated future" (1982: 207). Bruner (1986) states that the narration often involves two relational aspects: first, the narrator organizes experience both for another and for himself or herself at the same time; second, the narrator involves others as active listeners. Clark (1995) alludes to the effects of sympathy through sharing narration of suffering from losing human rights and respect.

Coles and Coles (1978: 232) state that the unhappy and complaining woman begins to move her attention from the individual or idiosyncratic to the broader arc of humanity and psychological indefiniteness by telling stories. A closer connection to a spouse was associated with decreased depressive symptoms for women. Spouse mutual closeness was associated with significantly decreased feelings of helplessness in wives (Tower and Kasl, 1996).

Korte (1979) suggested that, to study an elderly minority group, the researcher should elicit and interpret values, attitudes, norms about demeanor and difference, sentiments, worldviews and traditions, culture, and the history of the individuals or groups. To achieve this, case studies with life stories and explanations of health and illness experiences can be created. The evidence of individual variability within the elderly community is vital and tends not to portray aging as being uniformly positive (Luborsky, 1995: 278). The cultural, ethnic, or personal diversity in ideals or capacities of elderly people may need to be considered, especially in light of individual lifelong inequalities in health and social interdependency in old age, instead of focusing on individual competence and effort. "Anthropological interest in gerontology must illuminate aging and culture in a broad sense as well as provide humanizing and particularizing perspectives needed to counterweight the generalizing and reductionist view of social life in biomedicine" (Luborsky, 1995: 278). Both particularization of individuals with their groups (family) and generalization about a population's sociocultural health should be applied in order to understand the adaptive process.

To preserve the vivid natural expression of each informant about life and illness, I present the narratives as each one told them. I tried to translate them as closely as I could to convey what they said and meant. There are variations in lifestyles and expressions in the individual stories, although the informants have common life experiences: family, aging, immigration, self-awareness, and illnesses. The workings and interactions of common life experiences manifest and express different and various patterns, sounds, and colors.

Comments and interpretations were added to each story. The informants did not usually use "I," the first person pronoun, as they responded in Korean. However, in the English translation "I" was used to indicate the first person pronoun. Otherwise, it would not be clear whether the first person or the second person pronoun was meant when "I" was omitted. "I" may be related to individualism. "I" is usually said directly in America, but Koreans talk without using "I" unless they have to be specific.

It might be meaningful to analyze data as much as possible according to sociopsychodemographic variables such as age, gender, socioeconomic status, kinds of religion, and types of personality. The relationships between these sociopsychodemographic variables and the patterns of symptom presentation and self-care are drawn. It seems to be important to hear the indigenous explanations of the elderly informants about how they get ill and how they get better in a holistic sense. How do they express emotions? How do they explain degrees or types of emotion? We tried to understand by actively listening and interpreting their explanation, healing, and prevention of their illnesses, and how they explain their illnesses and live with them or cure them in their cultural context.

What makes Koreans happy or sad? Is it something within them or something or someone external? When do Korean elders have peace of mind? Beyond current circumstances or situations, and according to their feeling and cognition based on their worldview, what influences or governs their souls or makes their lives meaningful and peaceful? The ways in which the elderly immigrants spoke were respected and presented in order to reflect what they are, what they think, how they think, and what they do as much as possible.

The qualitative interpretation of the narratives will be focused individually on each informant regardless of whether the informant had major depression. Part of the reason is that responses to some of the questions of the SKIGD between the two groups did not differ demonstrably. When the informants were asked if they were currently depressed, fourteen informants diagnosed as depressed and thirteen informants diagnosed as not depressed all answered yes. Adding to the diagnosis confusion, nineteen informants diagnosed as depressed and nineteen informants diagnosed as not depressed both answered no to the same question (Pang, 1995). The key data are the individual life histories, because DIS-III may not capture narrated details of life and illness history in a cultural context. The informants' explanatory models represent unique expressions of their lives.

PART II: KOREAN-AMERICAN STORIES

Chapter 3

Trying to Live As Americans Do

The stories in this chapter relate to the acculturation process and immigrant life as experienced by elderly Korean immigrants. The informants expressed their emotional and physical health status and coping strategies. Their relationship with their children continued to be important, although it is changing.

OPTIMISTIC START: "I DON'T SEE PEOPLE, ONLY CARS ON THE STREET"

Mr. Pak is sixty-three years old and has a college education. His family lives in Korea. He has lived in America for four months. Mr. Pak said:

> I don't feel bad. Although I feel lonesome sometimes, I feel good most of the time because I have interests, I can drive my car, and I have hope of living a second life in America. In Korea I would see people walking about, but here I only see cars on the streets. I can't have fun watching people here in America. There are handsome, beautiful, and ugly people to be seen but I don't see many of them at all. I play *badook* [a Korean game of strategy], billiards, and golf. I learn English. I meet with friends to drink and talk about politics and other topics.
>
> I am concerned about the conflict relationship between Korean immigrants and black people. Other than that I don't have any other concerns. Some Korean immigrants have small busi-

> nesses such as grocery stores in black neighborhoods. The Koreans' poor English is ridiculed. Some black people complain that Koreans don't treat them kindly and courteously. A Korean woman merchant shot a young black customer in her store because she thought the person was a thief. Some Korean merchants have been robbed and killed by black people. It was said that some black people are angry and hostile with Koreans because Koreans earn money from them but they do not contribute to the black community. Numerous goodwill activities have taken place to reconcile the black people to Korean immigrants. These include: scholarship programs, inviting black people to visit Korea, food distributions, parties, enhancing mutual cultural understanding by putting on plays or choirs together with black people, educational opportunities such as invitations to martial arts like tae kwon do, job training, and supervised recreational opportunities for young people.
>
> In Korea I had *hwabyung* and depression because I failed in business. There is no medicine to cure these conditions. The only thing I could do was to overcome the difficulties one by one with my willpower and develop courage to rise above them.

Mr. Pak seems to be in a typically euphoric state of mind in this early stage of his immigrant life. He sounds determined to start a new life, although he expressed some uneasiness about racial problems. He is getting to know American society by participating in social and recreational activities to acquire information and a support network.

He recalls that he had *hwabyung* and depression in Korea but he got rid of them with his willpower, a form of nonmedical self-care. Apparently, he resolved his distress by labeling his painful life experience as *hwabyung*. By this time, he may have forgotten his experience, because he did not go into detail about *hwabyung*. He may wish to forget it, not to recall it at this hopeful time. His *hwabyung* experience may have made him even stronger and more determined for his future than if he had not experienced it at all.

He is full of hope and expectation about a happy and fresh life in America. Obviously, he is full of wit and humor, with an optimistic personality. He might not have to rush to seek a job at all, but could take it easy and live on what he earned in Korea. He has raised and educated his children.

Mr. Pak is not a typical elderly Korean immigrant because he tries to live in America without depending on his children. He came to America by himself, leaving his family behind in Korea. Most elderly Korean immigrants are invited by their adult children to come to America. Usually, their children, grandchildren, daughter-in-law, or son-in-law come first and settle down and then invite their elderly parents to join them. The parents usually live with their children for several years after their arrival. Based on individual needs, the children are involved to varying degrees in their parents' welfare, whether they live together or not.

SAD BUT NOT DEPRESSED: "ARE WE BEGGARS OR HOUSEGUESTS IN AMERICA?"

An eighty-year-old, college-educated former school principal, who has been living for twenty years in America, has been feeling somewhat awkward and uneasy about depending on welfare for his own and his wife's living expenses. Mr. Yoon shared his situation, thoughts, and feelings:

> Our daughter invited us. She is a director of a hospital in America. My wife and I were well educated and both of us worked as school principals. My son-in-law is a professor of economics in one of the universities in America. We live in a senior citizen apartment. We live and eat for free. The U.S. government provides everything. We are thankful and feel that we don't deserve to receive what the government offers us. Some of us say it is a gift from God. But does God say that we can eat free without working? Are we beggars or houseguests in America?
>
> My son died in the line of duty while he was working as a military physician in Korea. His driver was drunk and a car accident occurred. My son was ready to come to America after passing an examination to study. My wife and I were very sad but not depressed. I cannot describe the sorrow exactly. He

> disappeared even before he blossomed. Sometimes I cry out loud. I use *ch'enyom* [accept and resolve distress] to overcome sadness. No one can console me because they don't know what I am going through. Religion was necessary for me to overcome the grief by myself. I pray for his happiness in the "other world." Time is the medicine to heal us. As time passes, our grief will become thin. I burned up our son's possessions because they reminded us of him. I tried to forget the tragedy as soon as possible for the sake of our other living children.

Mr. Yoon appears to be an honest, open, righteous, and sensible gentleman. He takes great pride in his children, who are well-educated and successful professionals. He described his experience of sadness. Realizing his son's public service to their country helped Mr. Yoon's family to relieve their grief by appreciating with pride their son's achievement and contribution. According to Mr. Yoon, the kind and the degree of pain experienced from the death of one's own child is felt in a unique way by each individual. He described his son's death as an enormous loss. Removing all his son's belongings helped him forget the loss, focus on his son's proud moments, and live for the rest of his children and for his spouse. These are self-help behaviors based on Korean beliefs and practices. Religion also helped the family to ease their grief, and they asked God to lead their deceased son to heavenly bliss. Mr. Yoon denied having depression, but admitted to sadness, differentiating between the two conditions.

It is known through recent contact that Mr. Yoon did not join the wave of those becoming U.S. citizens, although his wife did. Mr. Yoon sounded as though he was uneasy about receiving financial assistance from the U.S. government. He may feel that he does not deserve public assistance because he did not work in the United States. As a former educator, he might have felt ashamed to lean on the U.S. government. According to some informants, especially elderly men, becoming a U.S. citizen means a kind of betrayal of their motherland. Mr. Yoon appears to feel that his roots are in Korea. However, he lives in America with appreciation and gratitude. Some other informants said, "We were told that it is all right to receive U.S. assistance because our children have been paying taxes."

ACCEPTING CHILDREN'S ADAPTATION TO AMERICAN WAYS

Mr. Son, seventy-one, has a high school education and has lived for ten years in America. He was concerned about living harmoniously with his children and with African Americans.

> We shouldn't expect our children to live the way we want them to, in an old-fashioned way. We have to learn American customs and values, such as individualism. One of my friends who was a professor in Korea expected his grown children to live according to his ways, but his children didn't listen to him. He was furious and telephoned me almost every day about it. I told him to be patient and try to understand his children's position and attitude. I was in the same boat. His son and daughter-in-law don't speak with their parents and they live somewhere else by themselves. They don't give money to their parents and they don't respect their parents. In Korea, when we are old, we expect our children to support us.
>
> In America, my wife and I ran a store until five years ago. I should understand Americans, including African Americans, and be courteous and kind to them as our masters, because they are our customers. If you are hurt by others, you have to be patient. If I had had a gun, it would have become much more risky. Koreans are too greedy. Korean immigrants should give back 50 percent of their interests to the community. Koreans should realize that they are too greedy and share their profits with others.

The elderly Korean informants have begun to realize that they have to let their children to adapt to the American way of life. They recognize that they can no longer dictate the strict traditional filial ethics of Korea to their children. As the narrative describes, Korean elders instruct one another about their new values and practices. Mr. Son described how they should be cooperative, reciprocal, and harmonious with family members as well as with other ethnic groups.

THE TRANSFORMATION OF DESPAIR INTO HOPE

Reverend Hur is a sixty-one-year-old minister who lives in his own house. He was invited to come to America by his wife's family and has lived in the United States for ten years, working as a laborer before becoming a minister.

> I worked hard like an animal. I could not even listen to the daily news because I was too tired after working all day. I experienced racial discrimination at work and in the handling of traffic violations. I just behaved as a dead person or obeyed like a servant every day. I was sad and depressed. I regretted coming to America. I wasn't looking forward to another day. I lived with empty feelings and wasn't interested in anything. I only lived because I couldn't die. The inhuman conditions were hard for me to bear. I lost all my courage and I gave up any hope. It was like the Israelites were treated in Egypt. I wasted lots of time. I became very close to God through the hard experiences, though.
>
> In Korea, we were thrifty and tried to save, but here in America, it was hard to live even day to day from hand to mouth. We lived without hope for some time. When I came home, I just ate and slept and that was all. It was hard because my English was not fluent. I attempted suicide due to the combination of conflicts and the stress of life as an immigrant. Depression, I should say, is one of the most serious problems and a lot of immigrants are suffering from it like I did. *Hwabyung* is just another name for depression. *Hwabyung* causes *shingyungshayak* [neurasthenia]. I suffered from *shingyungshayak* in the form of neurotic gastrointestinal upset.
>
> I didn't come across a decent solution until I found the Bible. I just pray and live by what the Bible says. Now I spend my days with church work and reading books. Now I thank God for my immigration experience in America. It will become a good foundation for a meaningful life for me. Now that I depend on God, there will no longer be empty feelings and sadness in my life. I am very content with my church life.

> There should be some special task force at the government level that would provide new immigrants with necessary help. The cruel treatment of new immigrants from different cultural backgrounds is not right and there is something lacking in the immigration policy. I just don't understand why the United States accepts immigrants. In order to accept aliens in America, there should be some way to help immigrants to adapt themselves to the new environment. Discrimination won't be eliminated for good; the government authorities try to ensure that there is no discrimination, but in real life, the problem of discrimination is serious. In particular, we can witness discrimination at work or when stopped by the police for a traffic violation. This experience is common to most Korean immigrants.

Reverend Hur overcame various hardships in America. He now treasures the experiences because he learned much from them. However, there were moments when he was pessimistic and depressed with his life as an immigrant. He was familiar with Korean illnesses in relation to depression-producing situations that may also cause physical diseases. However, he was not identified as having major depression by DIS-III. He recognized that he suffered from *hwabyung* as well as *shingyungshayak* as a form of physical illness originating from psychosocial stresses.

Reverend Hur had a positive transformation similar to that experienced by many other immigrants. He believes that God has blessed him and his family. He used the idioms of Korean popular illnesses spontaneously as his therapeutic strategies.

STRESS CAUSED BY DISCRIMINATION

Mrs. Hyung is sixty-five years old. Her husband is a minister and she is a church pianist. She studied music in a university in Korea. Mrs. Hyung described the difficulties of immigrant life:

> We had a dry-cleaning business and I could feel the discrimination from some of the customers. It is hard for me to describe it. They were unkind and moody without special reasons. Some kind of subtle condescending air seemed to demand a master-

> servant relationship instead of a mutual, courteous, business relationship. Also, although I worked ten hours a day, it was hard to save money in America in contrast to Korea. Even though we accumulated a small sum of money by being thrifty, we were fearful of being investigated.
>
> When my youngest daughter was in junior high school, I couldn't be at home for her because of my cleaning job. It still bothers me, although she is doing well now. She is happily married and continues her graduate study in pharmacology.

Mrs. Hyung's perceptions of discrimination could be real or imagined because of possible uneasiness about adapting to American value orientations and cultural expectations and low self-esteem from being a recent immigrant in the service business. Some examples of the related factors might be language and cultural differences.

Mrs. Hyung, as a working mother, experienced the dilemma of child care in the nuclear family, which can be compared with the extended family situation. She might not have so many regrets if she had the assistance of the extended family, which is usually available in Korea.

HELPING CHILDREN AND PREPARING FOR THE CITIZENSHIP TEST AT THE SAME TIME

Mrs. Kang, seventy, is married, has a middle-school education, and has been living in America for eighteen years. She spoke seriously from her experience:

> It is a real living hell to prepare for the examination for citizenship in the United States and, at the same time, help the children by running our four households. Do I have to take the citizenship examination? Is there any way I can avoid that? I had gout in my hip because I worried too much as I was preparing for the examination. I buy groceries and cook for four families: my two daughters, my grandson, and my husband. One of them would say, "We need a big jar of *kimchi*" [pickled vegetables] and the other would say, "We need a kettle of ox-tail or seaweed

> soup or oiled, salted, roasted seaweed." My daughter runs a grocery store. She and her husband have to leave for work before dawn and they come home late at night. They see the stars in the sky when they go to work in the morning and they see the stars in the sky when they come home at night. Our adult children have their own children too. They don't even have time to do their laundry. That is why I have to help them although I am busy preparing myself for the examination. I have to help them no matter how busy I am because of the examination, you know. My daughters who live in Korea can travel all over America to show and educate their children, but my daughter in the United States cannot do that although she lives right here in America. She is really busy and leading a hard life.
>
> My husband told me not to bother with the citizenship examination because he passed it and he could support me. For a while I didn't worry and the hip gout disappeared. But I started to study again. Is there any good, efficient way to pass the examination?

Although some parents and their children do not follow the traditional relationship, Mrs. Kang's highest priority is her children's welfare. She gives unconditionally to her family without expecting to receive anything in return. Although the citizenship examination is vital to her monthly income and housing, she didn't give up helping her children. It was extraordinarily stressful for her to prepare for the examination and to help her children at the same time. She feels this stress caused gout in her hip. The disease may be related to biopsychosocial stress. In Korea there are sayings such as: "A parent can take care of ten children but ten children cannot support one parent" or "Love goes downward but not upward." In other words, it is natural for parents to love their children and to make enormous sacrifices to help them, but children may not understand and show the same degree of love to their parents. In the past as well as in the present, children usually tend to take this love for granted. Almost all the informants seem to love their children as Mrs. Kang does: unconditionally, dutifully, patiently, and truly without flagging.

AN ELDERLY IMMIGRANT WOMAN'S LIFE

Mrs. Sym, a seventy-six-year-old married Catholic without a formal education, lived with her daughter for four years, helping with babysitting, cooking, and housekeeping until she moved to a senior citizen apartment with her husband. She has lived in America for fifteen years.

> Our daily life is so-so because we have enough to eat so that we don't feel hungry. We don't have "feet" [transportation] and don't speak English. I feel like I am a cripple. I am low-spirited. It is a big illness. There seems to be no solution. In a way we are used to our problems since we have lived here for more than ten years. We are fearful of ailments. Coming down with pain is like a thunderbolt. One of our children lives out of town and the other lives also quite a distance from us. It is hard to get hold of them, particularly when we have an emergency. We usually end up calling an ambulance or the family doctor and we let our children know later. At first, it was all right when we lived with our daughter. But now our grandchildren are grown up and our son-in-law is a stranger to us. We felt uncomfortable with him, so we moved out. Often we are lonely. We listen to the radio, watch Korean videos, and read Korean newspapers. We go to a "university" for elderly Korean immigrants because transportation is provided.
>
> My husband has been suffering from heart disease because he was cheated and lost all our money in a business deal. There was something hard in his chest and his heartbeats are fast. He had heart disease. He was so shocked, his vital energy was blocked, and he had a stroke. At first, he took medication but it got worse, and then he had surgery. My husband was very ill. His kidneys didn't work and he has been getting kidney dialysis. He didn't go to a hospital again and his condition got worse.

Mrs. Sym appreciates that her basic needs, such as food, are met. She said she is used to coping with language and transportation difficulties although she neither speaks English nor drives a car. For example, she speaks mainly Korean and depends on someone else for English. She does not own a car but depends on others (children, taxi, or friends) or public transportation. The most fearful thing for Mrs. Sym is facing emergency health problems, but she has learned to manage without her children's assistance by using medical services. Inevitably, she and her husband must live independently from their children. For Mrs. Sym, the sense of helplessness and powerlessness leads to loneliness. These feelings are experienced as a serious illness.

Mrs. Sym's explanation of her husband's heart and kidney diseases is related to social, moral, and ethical issues. She interpreted the health problems as a blockage of vital energy, which is grounded in Korean traditional medical principles.

Some Korean elderly immigrants seek all sorts of individual, community, or public resources to avoid burdening their children and to be independent from them as much as possible. However, the majority of Korean elderly immigrants look to their children for help first.

Chapter 4

Still Living by Korean Customs

The stories presented in this chapter relate to traditional Korean values, customs, and efforts at harmonizing and how they affect the lives of elderly Korean immigrants.

ANCESTOR VENERATION AND HWABYUNG: *PSYCHOSOCIAL, COSMOLOGICAL, AND SUPERNATURAL CAUSES*

Mrs. Sene, a seventy-six-year-old widow without a formal education, has been living in America for eight years. There are different stories about the causes of Mrs. Sene's *hwabyung*. This is her version. Her in-laws were making and spreading bad rumors about her without any grounds, which upset her. Mrs. Sene leans on her divorced daughter, without being able to solve any of her daughter's problems, or give her any help. She feels that she is only an additional burden to her daughter.

Mrs. Sene's daughter's version of the cause of Mrs. Sene's *hwabyung* is that her mother heard that if a ceremony to venerate their ancestors is held by the second son's family instead of the elder son's, they will be punished by their ancestral spirits. Being the wife of the second son in her husband's extended family, Mrs. Sene did not want to hold the ceremony, but had no way of avoiding it. She had to obey her elder sister-in-law (the first son's wife), who is next to the mother-in-law in the line of authority. Thus, she got sick psychogenically whenever she had to prepare for and perform the ceremony for her in-laws' ancestor veneration, which is rooted in Confucianism and shamanism.

The idea of ancestral punishment originated from clashes between two incongruent beliefs and practices, probably related to family conflict. Mrs. Sene added to what her daughter said: "If I could overcome everything worrisome, I would be fine, but I cannot." She felt powerless to refuse to perform the ceremony, although it was against her beliefs and practices. Mrs. Sene expressed tremendous anxiety and fear of offending the sacred realm she believed in. But she felt she should obey the Confucian principles of seniority (Chung, 1995). According to her upbringing, any slight hint of self-assertion and questioning of age, status, and hierarchy by women was frowned upon.

Mrs. Sene might have suffered from resentment and anger about being pressed to take over the elder son's wife's family ancestral responsibility. She did not voice this directly, but expressed her desperation in trying to avoid the responsibility related to the supernatural authority in a culturally appropriate manner. A supernatural explanation could be effective in making others understand why she did not want to take the responsibility. She must be a very traditionally oriented person and it might be very important for her to conform meticulously to Korean traditional ethics, morals, etiquette, and rituals to achieve harmony, respect, dignity, and satisfaction in life.

Psychosocial, cosmological, and supernatural beliefs affected Mrs. Sene and caused her to suffer from *hwabyung*. Fear of offending a supernatural being and possible retaliation for disobeying the commandments of the ancestor spirits seemed to cause Mrs. Sene's major emotional distress. The ceremony for ancestor veneration should be performed strictly according to rituals, etiquette, rules, and protocols (Janelli and Janelli, 1982). If not, the ancestors may retaliate against the offspring. Ancestors may not protect their offspring. The etiology of Mrs. Sene's *hwabyung* could have been compounded by current and past problems such as concerns for her daughter, interpersonal problems, and a fear of ancestral wrath.

Mrs. Sene's symptoms of *hwabyung* were anorexia, insomnia, feelings of suffocation, feelings of impending insanity and death, irritability, and loss of interest in normal activities. Mrs. Sene commented on the severity of *hwabyung*:

> I felt like I had become insane. The earth and the sky were falling down. I knew it was *hwabyung* because suddenly I got suffocating feelings and I felt a lump pushing up. I was afraid to be alone. It was severe enough to die. I followed my daughter wherever she went. I was afraid to be alone because I did not know what to do if those symptoms should come back. If it persists, death will follow because one cannot eat.

She was thankful to the interviewer who was listening to her and at the same time she said, "I am ashamed of telling you all my family stories." She complained of both physical and emotional symptoms. The symptoms of severe anxiety appeared to be a state of panic. Mrs. Sene expressed helplessness, a sense of insecurity, fearfulness, confusion, and depression. She also complained of a lump, a typical symptom of Korean illnesses. Mrs. Sene diagnosed herself as having *hwabyung* mainly based on feeling a lump. She believes that *hwabyung* becomes *shingyungshayak.*

Mrs. Sene said, "I knew I had to pray but I did not feel able to move even one of my fingers." She continued: "One should not be selfish but generous and understanding. We have to pray. I have a weak mind. I know that I have to overcome desires and hardships but I cannot overcome them. That is why it becomes an illness." She seems to be too sick to practice faith healing actively, although she believes in it. She did not come up with other self-care measures or coping mechanisms. Not having self-care or other methods could be considered a risk factor for Korean illnesses. However, people are energized by such illnesses, and those who are familiar with the Korean cultural context seek therapy through talking and listening with care for promoting understanding, sharing, and receiving *chong*.

A VIRTUOUS WOMAN LEADING A CONTENTED LIFE

Mrs. Gyung is a seventy-eight-year-old widow with a primary-school education who has been living in America for eighteen years. She is now living alone in a senior citizen apartment. She has three sons and one daughter. She is a Christian.

I live comfortably and pleasantly. I do not have any particular concerns. I don't want for anything. My children established the foundation for me to live in America. I am in good health. I have some communication problems, but I say, "Yes," "No," or "OK," and it seems to be working for me. When I cannot express myself, my children interpret for me. There is no one to really force me to speak English. I do not feel that I have wanted for anything. It is comfortable for me to live because I am used to living here now. I am not an intelligent, refined, and sophisticated person, so I just live during the day and sleep at night. That is all.

My eldest son has a doctoral degree and teaches in a university in America. He invited me to come to America. He told me that I could live anywhere I like, in Korea or America. I came to America in 1973 and started to care for my third son's children. When I finished raising my grandchildren with great care for ten years, I started to live in this apartment. When I was young, I worked hard around the house. It was good to live with my son and daughter-in-law. Now, I enjoy living in this apartment because I am old and do not have any work to do for my children. My son said, "Please live anywhere you like, in our house or in a separate apartment." I thought the offer was very reasonable and I moved into this apartment and I live by myself.

I have never quarreled with my son or daughter-in-law because they are both good people. I help my children whenever they are busy and they need me, and when they are not busy, I live my own life in this apartment. I do not know loneliness and I have not experienced loneliness because my grandchildren were great to me and I loved them. I believe in Jesus and I leave everything to God.

I was in good health in Korea. I took part in church life faithfully. I had gallbladder surgery in America. I am taking medicine for my heart and high blood pressure.

In Korea, my husband passed away early when I was only thirty-five years old. I earned my living expenses and sent three of our children to study in America. I had some hardships because I was the only one to earn a living in my family when my children were young. I had all sorts of small businesses. But still we were poor. Of course, at times I showed my worry about our future by saying, "How can I live with our children without their father?" My brother-in-law was helping us by visiting us and paying some tuition for our children.

We were living patiently and joyfully with hope. If you live joyously, good things happen. I have not given up anything. If you let yourself feel sad or depressed, unhappy things happen. I do my best and leave the rest to God. I read the Bible, sing hymns, and pray. I forget all unpleasant things. I knew I needed to love my children more than usual because they did not have their father, and I cared for them as best I could. My children are very kind to me, too. Also, I told my children to do their best. Up to now, I do not know how to complain because I have never complained. I did not feel lonely or have suicidal thoughts. Everyday I lived joyously. I did not complain even once to my son and, of course, to my daughter-in-law. I was a happy woman because our children studied very well. I didn't need to complain. It is no use to cry or to get frustrated or irritable. If you start having anxiety once, it will soon double.

Depression and sadness are also called *hwabyung*. I have not been depressed, sad, or lonely. I may be an idiot. I think I am lucky that way. It is a blessing from the Lord. I am not even the most faithful Christian. I just did my best. That is all. I obeyed the Church rules and offered to do my best. Then, I was blessed. When sad times arrived, I was not sad. Isn't it a blessing? I overcome everything with my Christian faith.

How can I, an ignorant person, dare talk to you about this and that? Living happily seems to be the most important thing. Thank you for coming and for helping.

Although Mrs. Gyung recognizes her hardships, she humbly minimizes them based on her self-cultivation. She is a religious, spiritual, and virtuous woman in the Korean tradition. She emphasizes a broad sense of harmony with others instead of only self-interest. She gives credit to her children for their harmonious relationships and life achievements but not to herself. She shows *oe yu na gang* (strong, strictly disciplined self, outwardly generous, and understanding others). Besides earning her living and raising her children, she worked as a volunteer through her church. She believes that she is leading a meaningful life and she is satisfied with it and thankful for it. She is able to lead a contented life although she does not speak English. Speaking English is not essential for a harmonious and contented life in America for her. She does not set her expectations unrealistically high, but seeks available and useful resources instead. She seeks simplicity in her life and appreciates it. She can do a lot with meager, basic resources. Others might demand many things or do something about it while Mrs. Gyung might settle for something less. She can have high levels of satisfaction with resources that would seem minimal to others, but which can be treasures to her. She feels that she is fortunate as she is. She repeatedly said that she has not experienced depression, sadness, or loneliness or any folk illnesses currently or in the past. She attributes her faith and blessed life to God. Her children gave meaning to her life and her children helped her to persevere in all her tribulations in her widowhood.

She is able to regulate her emotions and her cultivated character strengthens her even further. Some of the factors contributing to her contented life are: her religious faith; her flexible, accommodating personality; her children's understanding and success; and support from her children and from a relative. Also, her values and beliefs regarding the Korean woman as a wise, loving, faithful mother, loyal wife, and generous neighbor gave her a sense of dignity and esteem. There were no narratives of her embodiment of distress. The freedom and independence with flexible support and love from her children, and her spiritual and religious life do seem to give her peace, strength, and contentment.

When it comes to interpersonal relationships, she might not complain, but she willingly tolerates disadvantages for someone else's sake in order to create a high level of harmony, even though others might have treated her unjustly in her difficult, widowed life. In her family there might have been some disagreements as in other families, but she did not complain, criticize, or demand anything for herself in order to gain compliments from her family members and friends.

A CULTIVATED PERSON WILL NOT BE DEPRESSED

Mrs. Noh is a seventy-two-year-old widow with a primary-school education who has lived in America for ten years. She explained about depression through her own and others' experiences:

> People who have too much time, being too comfortable, and having leisure, sink themselves in their thoughts and slide into depression. It all depends on their personality. Letting themselves sink into sadness and depression depends on their personality and character. I heard that an elderly Korean cried when looking out through windows and others fainted during baby-sitting. To me, it all depends on how one governs one's own mind. It is from being narrow-minded—selfish, in other words—and one's inner illness is being pushed up.
>
> A passive person can be led to illnesses such as depression or *shingyungshayak.* It is up to one's mind. If a person is not joyful or lighthearted, he or she explodes with anger and gets restless, irritated, sick, and frustrated. Also, the person is bothersome, unreasonable, and annoying to others. Some people cannot overcome their tempers, and get sick and lie down with their head tied with a band to relieve headaches by putting pressure on it. If one's inner illness becomes severe, the person collapses completely. The pattern of illness is different from person to person. Fear shows that a person cannot govern one's own inner turmoil. All rise up from the mind. Unless a person has a congenital illness, it all depends on how one thinks critically and manages.
>
> One has to live with a peaceful mind and work. If one leads a busy life, she is bound to forget all worries, conflicts, and distresses. In life there are joys and hardships. When my husband died rather young, I didn't express or show any signs of my hopeless feelings in front of my children, although it was painful inside of me to endure. I don't think I experienced unbearable hardships as others did. My character might be described as harmonious and peaceful. I don't have much to be angry or frustrated about. There is peace in my family. Family disharmony seems to be the cause of *hwabyung*. In my life, there were times I shouted out of exploded fire and I was

> worried and depressed. Afterward I bore it all with patience and silence. When others cannot control situations such as parents-in-law and daughter-in-law or family disharmony, they tend to succumb to nerves [worries], *shingyungshayak,* and ultimately *han* and *hwabyung.*
>
> It would be ideal if one gets angry and it is all temporary. We are bound to live with frustrations and absurdity. We can't avoid them as long as we live in this world. My friends seem to be in the same boat on that. My greatest and unique joy is to see my God. There seem to be people who are too smart and sharp but they seem to be defeated by their arrogance.

Mrs. Noh believes that one who has a disciplined mind will never be bothered by depression. She identifies herself as a cultivated and disciplined person, she is not bothered by depression, and she ultimately attributes her strength of mind to God. Mrs. Noh asserts that wellness and a healthy mind can promote health and prevent and heal illness and diseases—beliefs found in Korean culture, everyday life, philosophy, and religion.

A WISE MOTHER AND A GOOD WIFE (HYUN MO YANG CHUH)

Mrs. Sung, an eighty-year-old widow with a grade-school education, raised and educated her five children to the highest level and took care of her bedridden husband for fifteen years. She had depression, *hwabyung,* and *shingyungshayak.*

> I had no choice but to come to America to baby-sit for my daughter, who lives alone after her divorce, although I couldn't speak English and didn't have transportation. I feel like I live in a prison without bars. My daughter was married to a bad gambler and womanizer. That is why she divorced her husband and came to America to avoid him. These kinds of things like divorce happen fatalistically. What can you do, because it is her fate? Because my daughter is pitiful, I cried every day, hiding it from my daughter-in-law. I really wish to see my daughter living happily again with a good husband.

I worry and feel sad, especially when family members do not tell me when they are sick. When I feel lonely after my daughter and grandson leave for work and school, I miss Korea. I take a walk for about half an hour, then I feel good. I prepare supper and help my grandson with his homework.

I had hardships and used *shingyung* [worries] too much in my youth, and then I became weakened. I educated five children to the highest level without anybody's help. I told my children, "If you do not study now, you may lose your chance for education forever." I skipped meals and tightened my belt because there was not enough to eat. I wanted to give my children even a little more instead of eating it myself. When I look back I had a hard time. I believe that education is the most important thing and did my best to educate my children, although it was very hard. As a result, all my daughters and daughters-in-laws are devoted children. I think they appreciate my hard work for them. Also, I took care of my bedridden husband, who suffered with a stroke, for fifteen years, from when I was thirty-nine. He passed away at age fifty-four. I wish that he had lived at least to sixty for my children's sake.

I cannot sleep and I have hearing problems and backaches. I use a magnetic belt for backaches all the time. I went to a doctor. He said it is an old person's illness and it is related to the hardships I experienced in the past. I had injections, Korean traditional medicine, and Western medicine, but I don't think the backaches will be better.

On top of these problems, others cheated me out of my money. I had *hwabyung* and *shingyungshayak* for thirty years, until I was seventy years old. Sometimes I had these illnesses three to five times a day. By the time I was eighty years old, the illnesses had all disappeared.

When I was thirty-nine, my husband was bedridden, my small business was bad. Our house was burned up during the Korean War. My youngest child was two years old. How can I tell you all the hardships I went through? I felt that heaven was destroyed and earth was sunken. Now I have forgotten everything since it is over. When my sons distinguished themselves, all my worries disappeared.

> I pushed all the unpurified poisonous emotions deep down in the bottom of my mind. A physician advised me to do so. If I am angry or worried somehow or having conflicts, it will disappear soon by my inner digestion of distress. These days I do not "use nerves" [worrying] much.
>
> After my husband's death, I could come to America. If he had not died, how could I have come? I should have taken care of him. Besides, I helped all my children to get married. After that, I didn't have anything to do. So I could come to America and go back to Korea as I want.
>
> I have several daughters-in-law, and it made me feel better sometimes. However, daughter-in-law and daughter are different from one another. No matter how well a daughter-in-law treats her mother-in-law and how good and kind she is to her mother-in-law, the mother-in-law has to be careful because she is the daughter-in-law, not her own daughter. I can do whatever I want with my daughter but not with my daughter-in-law.
>
> My sons are very good to me. But, still I am a little lonely here in America. I receive Medicare, food stamps, and Supplemental Security Income (SSI). I really do not have anything to worry about or fear. I am old. I brought up all my children. My biggest worry was to bring up my children correctly. I was depressed then but not now. I love to go out with my children to dine out or to do something with them.
>
> Medication does not cure depression, but one has to learn to think right and be flexible by self-cultivation and be reasonable and understanding, breathe fresh air, eat good food, and work hard. I taught my five children to live actively and happily.

Mrs. Sung seemed to be able to maintain her sanity through her children's success, support from her children and relatives, taking an active role in her family, her outgoing personality, and mental self-care. Generally, she is satisfied with her life, although she is concerned about her divorced daughter. She seems to identify depression, *hwabyung,* and *shingyungshayak* as the same illness and gave the same explanatory models for them.

Mrs. Sung diagnosed herself as having *hwabyung* and *shingyungshayak.* She had to experience *hwabyung* and *shingyungshayak* to become a *hyun mo yang chuh* (a wise mother and a good wife). It was worth it to have suffered *hwabyung* and *shingyungshayak* because she made a *hyun mo yang chuh* of herself. *Hwabyung* could be considered a symbol of perseverance in honorably meeting the hardest challenges. She was not immune to *hwabyung* and *shingyungshayak*, although she is open, sensible, generous, and cultivated. To Mrs. Sung, it is not a stigma to have these illnesses but an honor because it takes many hardships to be recognized as a *hyun mo yang chuh* by herself, her own children, her in-laws, and others.

Generally, human relationships might be more complex in Korea than in America; it may be related to collectivism versus individualism. Mrs. Sung enjoys compatibility with others, for example, with her daughter, but she proved that she could get along with everyone including her daughter-in-law, although she clearly distinguishes her daughter from her daughter-in-law in terms of relationship factors such as level of mutual comfort, dependability, reliability, caring, etc.

Mrs. Sung said that she wished her children's father could have lived longer for her children's sake. She expressed it this way because it is the accepted fashion of communication as *hyun mo yang chuh*, although she herself also truly wished her husband had had a long life. In her time, marriage was intended to continue the patriarchal lineage, not for romance. A woman's role and function in marriage are mainly to aid in the creation of offspring. Thus, language and custom reflect the patriarchal orientation.

Now she is approaching ninety years of age. She is pretty much disengaged from worldly matters and, consequently, she is free from the illnesses that she constructed based on her hardships.

She demonstrated that perpetual, harmonious, caring, and nurturing human support is the most important healing process, in her holistic explanatory model, including her pluralistic medical practice.

LIVING IN A FOUR-GENERATION EXTENDED FAMILY HOUSEHOLD

Mrs. Um is a sixty-seven-year-old married Christian with a grade-school education who lives with her husband and mother-in-law. She willingly and openly shared what has been going on in her life:

We came to America in 1981. I worked in a sewing factory and my husband cleaned buildings. We moved out here to live so that we can avoid the conflicts of living with our children. My illness recurred because it was so hard for me while I was taking care of my grandchildren, who were one year apart. I used to have insomnia, vomiting, and dizziness related to my son's death. I had *shingyungshayak.* Now, I am fine after moving out and living here away from our children. In general, my husband and mother-in-law supported me.

Yes, I had tribulations and trials in my life. My husband was forced to become a student soldier by the Japanese and we were separated from each other for a year and a half. He came back after the Korean independence from the Japanese occupation. My husband joined the army during the Korean War. My father-in-law was killed in the bombing. It was very hard not knowing whether my husband was alive or not. In Korea I blindly obeyed my parents-in-law, husband and family members, so much so that I had headaches and indigestion and a lot of nerve-related illnesses [worry, conflicts, or distress].

I lost my infant son. My first son died of measles. I felt something like a lump in my chest and it lasted for a year. My chest was painful. Every day, for a while, I experienced a vision or illusion or hallucination that my dead son was crawling in my room. Sometimes I was fearful to enter my room because I felt like my son was lying there. I was fearful because I was overwhelmed with my sorrow. I was worse after his funeral was over. How could I even cry when I was attending to my mother-in-law, a senior elder of our family? The death of my son is not a proud matter. I cried alone only at night. Neither could I share my sadness with my husband nor with my mother-in-law, who believe in digesting one's inner turmoil within and alone. I didn't think they understood what I was going through and what I was experiencing. I could not sleep and I contracted *shingyungshayak* and depression because my soul was painful and sad. I was depressed for a year. I was able to overcome the agony, the hopelessness and helplessness, by myself. It was a mind illness, so there was a cure. I had my second son and I became attached

> to him with love. I was able to overcome the sadness from my first son's death.
>
> However, these days I am concerned and somewhat depressed about my later life.
>
> In America, I have peace of mind because my husband has been faithful to me. Lately I can tell my husband whatever I want, although we have differences of opinion sometimes. It helps my mental health. However, I still have to be restrained in front of my mother-in-law so that at night I am very fatigued and ill, because I am the sort of person who is very patient and works hard to be perfect.

The distress of her infant son's death, the restraint necessary to live with a ninety-year-old mother-in-law, the worry of her husband's potential desertion related to her low educational status, and her worries for her husband during the Japanese occupation and the Korean War have caused Mrs. Um much *shingyung* (concerns, emotional burdens, oversensitiveness or worries) throughout her life.

When Mrs. Um was young, she suffered extremely from the loss of her son. She admitted that it was even harder to endure it all by herself. If she could have worked it out with others such as her husband, it would not have been so hard. There is a strong belief in Korea that if something is wrong with a child's birth or rearing, including having a girl instead of a boy (boys are preferred in patriarchal Korea) or being unable to bear a child, it is considered the wife's fault. It is hard for a wife to expect to be consoled in this situation. The sense of being understood and cared for one's by family is not always guaranteed to daughters-in-law in Korea. Mrs. Um was lonely even in her extended family. In other words, she felt alienated. In traditional Korea, a barren woman is sent back to her parents' home. She did not expect her mother-in-law to sympathize with her because it is expected that the mother-in-law will think that there is something wrong with her daughter-in-law. Thus, she could not even cry in front of her mother-in-law and husband because they might think or say, "Why does she cry all the time? She should be ashamed of herself that she lost her child because she didn't do her best in taking care of her child. And she might not deserve a son."

Also, it is likely that her mother-in-law and her husband were grieving and mourning inwardly as much as Mrs. Um, but they did not express it outwardly because they learned to restrain their emotional pains and sorrows. A man is not expected to express feelings of dignity and respect, but to be stoic, serving as a role model to stabilize the family emotionally. The same might be true for Mrs. Um's mother-in-law as the matriarch of the family.

Mrs. Um was tired mentally and physically from looking after her mother-in-law and her grandchildren in her old age. She had to display formal, ritualized behaviors in speaking, sitting, interacting, and caring for all the needs of the matriarch of her household. Both mother-in-law and daughter-in-law are familiar with traditional Korean customs because both of them, almost as a team, learned and lived in the traditional Korean value system. Mrs. Um treats her mother-in-law formally. Perhaps she knows that her mother-in-law may be more comfortable with traditional ways, and most of all she expects and anticipates from her daughter-in-law the traditional formal way of support. In Korea or America, for the elderly mother-in-law, a daughter-in-law is a daughter-in-law whether she is young or old.

Mrs. Um believes that illness based in the mind is curable because the mind depends on the person's cultivation, disposition, emotions, will, determination, and regulation. To Mrs. Um, mind and emotions are malleable. One can make oneself happy or unhappy. In Mrs. Um's case, her own positive, individual mindset as well as a less hierarchical, lenient, and relaxed relationship with her husband helped her have a somewhat peaceful mind in America.

DEALING WITH AGE DISCRIMINATION

Sixty-seven-year-old Mr. Un, with a vocational-school education, has lived in America for ten years.

> I have memory loss and financial difficulty. I have a problem supporting my ninety-year-old mother. I can move to a senior citizen apartment after my mother passes away. I was lonely right after immigrating. I could not speak English and I did not have friends. I missed my children very much. I began to feel

better as my children began to reunite with us one by one from Korea. And my work as a cleaning person helped me to overcome the unbearable loneliness. Now, after my retirement, I work in my children's gardens, cutting the lawn and things like that. I go around to my children's homes one by one to look after them with this and that.

In order to educate my seven children in Korea, I did not even have time to be ill or feel good or bad. I enjoyed working in a bank as a manager and handling currency. That was a good job. However, Korea is a hierarchical society. They discriminated against me because of my age. They tried to get me to quit. Finally I resigned. I had a hard time with the supervisors.

I was outraged and sad because I was treated as an old man despite my young mind. I was suffering from the thought of giving up my life. Psychogenic duodenitis developed at this time. I was bothered by vomiting. My face turned a dark color and I could not sleep. *Hwabyung* developed due to the momentary shock of the forced resignation and consequent mental and physical agony, and lasted for two to three years. The illness occurred every three to four months at the time of seasonal change.

I was depressed every day for a year and a half. I had empty feelings for several months after my resignation. I was severely depressed, enough to wish to die. I was pessimistic about prolonging and living my life. I just lived with the attitude that if somehow I didn't die I would live. The only thing I was worried about was my family. I almost gave up my life, whether to live or die. I learned that I couldn't take it easy and take time, but I shouldn't get easily frustrated and angered. I had to kill my acute fire and strong explosive emotion. I suffered all by myself. Nobody knew what I suffered from. My third daughter-in-law helped me as a tranquilizer. My wife could not help me because she had to work as a peddler. I did not experience any improvement from the hospital care I received. I just stay at home these days. I am careful about what I eat and I try to have peace of mind.

In Korea even people who work hard cannot survive. But, in America, if one works hard, he can be paid fairly for his work. I also had a hard time in the army during the Korean War.

Mr. Un expressed rage as something dangerous and alive and having the potential to ruin his status as a gentleman, so that he had to "kill" (relieve) it. He almost personified the rage as a dangerous person, who would surely harm him by causing disasters or at least making the situation worse. If he does not kill it, it will keep him from becoming a cultivated social being. Otherwise, he may be controlled by the emotion, and he may act out and go berserk. It will bring something worse to him than losing face in Korean society, such as losing his health.

Consequently, he suffered from depression and *hwabyung*. Actually, he described the same symptoms for depression and *hwabyung,* so that the illness he had could be called by either name. At the end of the third year after he resigned from work, he came to the United States. If he had not made this change, he might have committed suicide. His ability to accept the reality of his former work, environmental and occupational changes, diversions such as immigration, different ways of thinking and emotional control, and mutually caring relationships with his children helped him to alleviate the *hwabyung* and depression.

Mr. Un lives with his ninety-year-old mother, which can be considered traditional filial piety. At the same time, he takes care of his children, and his mother and children take care of him. The filial piety runs broad and deep. The phenomena of value change and continuity seem to depend on individuals and situations in the family and society. According to Mr. Un's experience, traditional family values such as filial piety and mutual caring seem to be continued longer than those of society. The status and respect due to elders might be recognized in Korea, but not their continued ability to function. Maybe the elderly must adhere to their assigned roles; for example, it probably is not acceptable to work continuously at an advanced age.

Chapter 5

Parents Can Take Care of Ten Children, but Ten Children Cannot Support Their Parents

The stories in this chapter deal with the relationships between the elderly Korean immigrants and their children and grandchildren in America and Korea. They show how socioeconomic, cultural, ethical, and moral combinations influence the mind, emotions, and the body.

LIVING INDEPENDENTLY AND TRANSCENDING GRIEF

Mrs. Im, eighty-six, is married, has a high school education, and has lived in America for fourteen years.

> I feel free because my husband and I live away from our children. When we were living together with our children, we didn't feel comfortable. In Korea, children consider old people useless. Old people are like a diseased tree standing up. The diseased tree falls down when the wind blows because it is empty inside. If nothing hits the tree, it will remain standing up. Old people need help from their children, but old people are afraid to signal the need for support, in case their children might be offended, or they are afraid that they might unexpectedly plant a seed of guilt in the heart of their children in case they cannot help them.

Mrs. Im depicted the vulnerability of elderly people by using natural phenomena and catastrophic forces as metaphors. Advanced age is characterized as a diseased state. Therefore, old people require support from their children.

Mrs. Im is concerned about her relationship with her children. Dependency, independence, and reciprocity between parents and children are frequently considered issues. Elderly parents are aware of the need to live independently from their children for mutual convenience. Some children are reluctant to live with their parents even though children are expected to be filial. Parents are aware of the possible necessity for independence and, therefore, they take the initiative. Deep down in their hearts, elderly parents want to live with their children with reasonable privacy, space, and flexibility, ideally under the same roof, so that they can be as independent as possible. Mrs. Im and her husband set up a separate household for more or less mutual convenience for their children and themselves. However, it was more for their children's convenience. Mrs. Im might have been somewhat ambivalent about the situation since she believed that she had health problems, and she would have liked to live with people who could give her care when needed.

Mrs. Im shared her personal and spiritual feelings, thoughts, and meanings:

> One of my sons died during a sports game and my younger daughter died of tuberculosis. Sometimes, if a young man runs around, I feel like my dead son is running to me and calling "Mother!" or opening the door to my house and coming in. When I see a young girl who sings well, I think: "She is my daughter." So much so that my elder daughter worried that I might have become insane. At that time I developed stomach spasms, which I didn't have before. I think all these phenomena occurred because I still love my children and I miss them so much. I am continuously very sad and feel sorry for myself. I think of Job from the Bible. I pray as I cry loudly. I cry because there is no other way to relieve my frustration with my helplessness. I pull myself up when I realize there is a God. One has to govern one's mind and comfort oneself. I think of my positive qualities. I reaffirm and strengthen my faith to go to heaven and meet my children there. I feel I have confided all my secrets to you.

Mrs. Im seems to have delayed resolving her grief and still mourns for her children, although their deaths occurred quite a long time ago. She seems to suffer from some phenomena of *han* and *shingyungshayak* as expressed in Korean terms. She was not identified as having major depression by DIS-III.

Mrs. Im seems to be on the way to healing. In her hope of uniting with her children in the afterlife, she is devoting herself to her spiritual life. This may relieve her feelings of shame or guilt that mothers commonly have, whether the pain of the loss is justified to others or not. The other healing strategy that Mrs. Im uses is to identify with Job from the Bible and take Job as her role model to create a meaningful and acceptable sense of self.

HAPPINESS AND GRATITUDE

Mrs. Turk is a seventy-eight-year-old widowed Christian with no formal education. She talked about her life:

> Good. It's fun. God gave us health. My children are all healthy and have good jobs. I don't have to deal with my daughter-in-law who doesn't agree with me here in America because she is in Korea. My son asked me to return to Korea. What can I do if I get sick in Korea? Here in America medical insurance pays for me. What can I do if I return to Korea and I don't like it? How can I come back? That's why I decided to stay right here in America. I really like my kitchen. How can I own a refrigerator in Korea if I have to move out to live in a small rented room because my daughter-in-law and I don't get along in Korea? In America, I don't have any problems except for language and transportation. I solve my problems through my children.

By living in America, Mrs. Turk was able to avoid poverty and the well-known, traditional, antagonistic relationship between mother-in-law and daughter-in-law. Mrs. Turk continued:

> After living two years with my daughter, I now live alone in a senior citizen apartment. I am just thankful because I am given

this place to live in, money, and medical care, although I have not done anything for America. The ambulance comes when we need it. I don't feel lonely. My children come and go and I see friends frequently, and we help each other. It is much better to live here than in my child's empty house after they have gone to work. I really like living in America. I became a citizen of the United States. I am really thankful. I look forward to going to church on Sundays. I see a lot of Koreans in my church so that I feel like I am in Korea. My children are required to pick up food stamps for me. I know it takes a lot of my children's time, so I told my children not to bother with those stamps.

My husband joined the army voluntarily in China and was killed in military action in 1940. It was very hard to live alone at that time. I raised my three children all by myself. During the Korean War, we escaped to my parents' home. My son-in-law died of leukemia, but all his children were educated. He studied in America because he believed that he had to become an "American." At that time I was sad and depressed. I had depression. I was about to become insane. I thought I'd better die than live a troubled life. I didn't want to meet people. It was severe. I wasn't interested in living. I couldn't sleep and couldn't eat. I just sighed. My family became chaotic.

But I didn't try to kill myself because committing suicide is sinful, and then I wouldn't be able to go to my Father's [God's] home. One day I thought I had to pull myself up. I leaned on my God. I overcame the misery with my faith. My depression disappeared. I prayed and read the Bible. I like God's words such as we shouldn't follow material pursuits, but His grace. Don't talk about others but keep your heart joyful. Just because I have worries inside, I make an ugly face, then I look ugly, and others cannot help me. I console myself and I always thank God. Then it is good because endorphin is released. In Proverbs, chapter 17:22, it says, "A cheerful heart is good medicine, but a downcast spirit dries up the bones." I am a joyful person and I like to work for my children.

We are on a diet. We eat unpolished rice and never eat meat. Abalone and shrimp contain the highest amount of cholesterol.

It is wonderful to know that a person can recover from depression after having hardships in life such as a spouse's early death, war, poverty, a son-in-law's death, and conflicts with a daughter-in-law. Because Mrs. Turk experienced hardships, it is possible for her to appreciate all kinds of support. She is deeply religious. According to her testimony, religion made her a healthy and positive person.

It has frequently been said that Korean elders who suffered from poverty in Korea appreciate living in America with welfare, but those who enjoyed a luxurious life in Korea do not appreciate America as much. Probably, they were made helpless and powerless because of the language difficulty, inconveniences from sociocultural differences, unfamiliarity with American life, the loss of friendship, and independence.

HWABYUNG *AND INTERGENERATIONAL CONFLICTS*

Mrs. Yi, a seventy-five-year-old widow with a middle-school education, was brought up on a farm. She has three children who are all highly educated. One of her sons died. She said, *"Na nun Bok I up nun sa ram iya"* (Happiness does not come to me as I deserve or wish).

> My life is very sorrowful. I think my illness is a nerve or psychogenic condition from my sadness. It is very sad to think of leaving this world, death. Children are useless because they are very busy. They cannot do anything for me. If I live with one of my children, my illness will be healed up right away. I lived with my daughter, but she wanted me to move out. None of my children tells me to live together with them. Actually, my youngest son invited me to live with his family, but I don't want to live there because my grandchildren don't speak Korean and, therefore, they don't like me. My daughter doesn't want me to live with her. I feel betrayed by my daughter. I am easily irritated and angry. My daughter does not want me to visit her either. My feelings of betrayal by my daughter are much greater than my distress at my husband's death when I was twenty-seven years old.

If I live with my daughter, I will be healed. My daughter was a filial daughter. However, since she has been living in America, she has changed. I don't know exactly what changed her. I was very sad and depressed when my daughter left this injury in my soul. Now her personality is cold and peculiar and she is not at all compassionate. Actually, she is a warm person but she speaks in a cold and insensitive way.

My daughter-in-law also doesn't like me. I live in a senior citizen apartment. I would feel better if I were allowed to live with someone. I do not have friends. I do not have the personality to make friends very well and stay close. Loneliness is my biggest pain. I was widowed when I was twenty-seven years old. When I was thirty-three, I remarried and bore my last son. But my second husband was a womanizer. So I departed and came to America.

I am a person with lots of *han*. If I take a tranquilizer, I feel a little better. I am longing for human compassion. I am sad constantly so that I'd rather die. My only consolation is writing my diary. Although I didn't have any financial problems, I injured my soul myself and provoked *hwabyung*. The shock I had when I left my daughter's place triggered the *hwabyung*. When I am depressed and sad, I feel dizzy right away in my head. Then I can't get up due to dizziness and it is really dark in front of my eyes. I was told that the blood capillaries in my brain were obstructed. I worried about having a stroke. According to my doctor, my backaches are from my nerves [worries, conflicts, and distresses] but I don't know much about it.

Even these days I cry because I am sad. I do not know why but I am always sad. In Korea I did not worry much. Since I came to America, I have more tears and illnesses. I suffer from homesickness. I think it is related to nerves. It is something to do with the pains in my mind. My sorrow becomes lumpy as well as watery and it comes out as tears. After ten years, my tears come down a little less. I cannot tell you how much I cried. I feel pressured in my mind and heart. Today I don't have depression and I just feel happy because I am talking with you like this. How good it is to talk openly. When I am depressed, I go out for a walk. Then I am all right.

> Recently I am doing better. I thought I would die without my daughter and I couldn't live without her. All the people I trusted left me and it made me very sad. My son died of liver cancer. I think I miss people more than other people would if they were in my situation. But actually now I feel even more comfortable than when I lived with my daughter. The passage of time is an efficacious medicine for me. I accepted some and gave up some, gave in some, and I am feeling better in my human relationships. My daughter and I go to the grocery store together these days. I participate in activities with other elderly American people, although I speak very little English. I communicate with gestures and by observations. There are only a few Koreans, so I have to get along with Americans. I do not go to church because my daughter is busy writing her autobiography and other things. She does not have time to give me a ride. I try to live happily. But that is not easy. How can I live happily when there are no happy events? Nobody visits me. I am just sad. I live because I cannot die.
>
> I had herbal medicine, acupuncture, and physical therapy. The physical therapy relieved my backaches. The other ones were not effective. To relieve depression one has to cultivate one's mind. Except for a peaceful soul, all the others are useless. My daughter does not want me to tell about my situation or what I think of her to others, and I have to try to digest my awful, distressing emotions inside myself.

Mrs. Yi blames her daughter, daughter-in-law, grandchildren, friends, and her lack of cultivation for her unhappiness and loneliness. She believed initially that the only way to happiness is to have someone else's support. The language difference between Mrs. Yi and her grandchildren has interfered with their relationship. Mrs. Yi seemed to feel guilty about criticizing her daughter, so she frequently said that her daughter is a warm person. Mrs. Yi may be ambivalent about her daughter. Directly and indirectly, Mrs. Yi admitted that the love from her children and her love for them is more precious than that which she received from her spouse.

Her daughter didn't grant her mother what she wanted, which was to live together. However, they reconciled and negotiated an agreement with some conditions. They live separately, but they know that they can still care for each other and do things together. Mrs. Yi found that there are ways to compromise. Finally, she seems to realize that happiness comes from within oneself somewhat. She no longer wishes to live with her daughter, but rather seeks ways to get along with American residents.

Mrs. Yi's construction of her illness appears to have a soul-body relation in connection with her perception of her daughter's betrayal, along with disharmonious relationships with her daughter-in-law and grandchildren. She relates her emotional distress (depression) to bodily symptoms such as backaches and a potential stroke. Her explanatory model shows that she embodies psychosocial origins of distress and relates them to her physical illnesses. Sometimes she takes medication. She seems to call the whole distressing mind-body relationship *hwabyung*. There is a Korean saying: *"gi sung ie myun gam chun"* (If you do your best, Heaven will be impressed with you and Heaven will help you). She believes ultimately in cultivating and strengthening the whole mind and soul to have peace of mind. She said, "It is up to how one thinks and carries it out. Brighten your soul and beautify yourself inside and outside. I make up and dress up and go out. It makes me feel wonderful."

When Mrs. Yi was contacted recently, her son was visiting her from Korea. However, she seemed to be able to lead her own life away from her children, and she appears to be close to some American residents. Now she seems to get along with everyone, including her family members, after coming a long way, although she can be fragile, labile, and vulnerable in certain stressful situations. It seems to have something to do with her insight about her life experience and nature's way.

DEMYSTIFYING FAMILY SOLIDARITY: "I FOUGHT WITH MY ONLY CHILD EVERY DAY"

Mrs. Sim is a seventy-six-year-old widow with no formal education.

> I have *shingyungshayak* because my daughter didn't treat me kindly and with respect. It is very difficult for my daughter and me to get along. The way she thinks and does things is quite

different from what I think and do. I fought with my only child every day. I ran away from my daughter's house and lost all my clothes during the chaos.

My daughter told me, "When you were well off, you did not give us anything. Why are you bothering my husband and me so much now that you have lost all your possessions?" My daughter and son-in-law resent me because they feel that I did not care for them when I was able to. Their grocery business is not booming. She shows her *hwapoori* [anger and resentment] by accusing and blaming me.

My daughter asked me to move out and live alone. She treats me horribly. She treats me as though I demand her support unreasonably and as though I were senile and had poor judgment. My daughter is authoritative enough to ask her own mother to act like a dead person or servant in front of her. I am not allowed to say anything or ask for anything, but should be obedient to her. If I had a place to move to, I would have done that already. I have been lonely until now. I was so helpless. I wanted to die. I attempted suicide but failed. I was about to take drugs as recently as two days ago. I fight every day, every hour with my daughter and grandchildren. My daughter was trying to persuade me to move out. Everybody claims that he or she is right in her family. I am the only one who is always wrong. I don't want to live like this even one more hour. I pray that I can move out. Then I imagine that I could live as I wish to and have fun with other elderly people in an apartment. I could buy and eat what I want to eat. I cry every day and I insist on going back to Korea but my daughter does not do anything about it.

Mrs. Sim elaborated further on her reasons for her suicide attempts:

If I say something, my grandchildren treat me as though a dog barks. They don't buy me what I want to eat. I cannot buy it myself because I don't have "feet" [transportation] in America. In Korea, I went everywhere I wanted to go and did everything. I went to market. I visited my friends and my friends came to visit me. Here my daughter doesn't want to let my

> friends visit me in her house. I just do housekeeping and lie down because I am not feeling well. My daughter's family says to me, "Do not eat watercress. It is very expensive." This makes me resentful and angry, but I try to be patient. It is not easy to control my anger. That's why it becomes *shingyung-shayak* [neurasthenia]. I use too much *shingyung* [thinking intensely to solve problems]. I lost all my possessions with monetary as well as sentimental value during the unsettled life situation. That is also one of the reasons for having *shingyung-shayak.*

Mrs. Sim expected her daughter's support, while her daughter is not caring toward her mother because she does not think she has received the maternal care and inheritance that she deserved. Mrs. Sim feels that she is not even respected as a human being. Not being treated with filial piety by her daughter is unthinkable for Mrs. Sim. Her daughter believes in mutual caring instead of giving or receiving one way. Also, the effects of acculturation influence their relationship. Traditional family positions in relation to respect, power, and authority have been switched between parents and children. The solidarity of intergenerational cooperation and caring has been diminished.

Mrs. Sim does not move around well and cannot do much housework. This situation makes her daughter nag her even more. Mrs. Sim said, "My emotions flare up and my emotions and hers clash with each other. I sigh and feel resentful about my poor life. I am just fixed on my past so that I don't look forward to my future. I sacrificed my life and lost my health. There is nobody who is as sick as I am." Mrs. Sim was disappointed with her daughter and she feels sorry for herself.

> I am bothered by my daughter every day. I try to be patient and then my headache develops. My crying means that I am silently trying to endure the insults from my daughter. My whole body aches. Due to the mental shock of my daughter's maltreatment, my mind and body are all diseased. I have *shing-yungtong* [nerve-related pains on buttocks, extremities, thighs, or neuralgia].

I "use nerve" [brooding, worries, distress, or stress] every day. I am depressed and the symptoms get worse. I go berserk and act out. Then I just think that I wish I could die. I lost my health and sacrificed all my life for my family. When my husband's business failed, I was sad. I don't think I had depression at that time but there were depressive symptoms. I lost confidence.

I had a son but he died young while still in middle school. During that difficult time, I lived with my sister. At that time I was beside myself. My soul ran out of me or escaped from my body— *hon be baek san* [astonished and terrified]. I was almost crazy.

Moving out of my daughter's house is the only solution. I am trying to find an apartment.

In order to endure my loneliness, I listened to music and I did knitting and sewing. Sometimes I covered myself all over with a thick blanket and slept in order to forget the loneliness. My sisters and brothers sympathized with me. I want to go back to Korea even now. It was good because I lived alone in Korea. I had many relatives and friends. I speak Korean. If I go to Korea, I feel all my illnesses and diseases will be cured. I think of the airplane that flies to Korea all the time. If I go to Korea, I don't have to suffer from the hell of living in conflict with my daughter. My "inside is rotting" [*Sok eul suk da*—a miserable feeling of decay and agonizing distress]. Others told me that all daughters are like that and they asked me to just be patient. I think all the elderly Korean people living in America live like I live.

Reciprocity or exchange of support seems very important to maintain mutually supportive relationships between parents and children in Korean families. Mrs. Sim stated that she is not the only one in such a situation, and it is rather common among the elderly Korean immigrants.

"Being depressed and sad is being injured inside" (*sok i sang ha da*—having anger, conflict and resentment), said Mrs. Sim. Emotional disturbance is expressed with a somatic idiom. It appears that, ultimately, Koreans seem to be concerned about body integrity being damaged by interpersonal, social, and environmental disharmony. In other words, from her experiences, she concluded that illness has a social origin.

When her daughter entered during the interview, Mrs. Sim suddenly said that she was having pains that caused her to feel as though she was dying. According to the mother, the daughter also complains about her sluggish business and other frustrations to her mother in an accusatory tone. There seemed to be no genuine or mutual caring relationship between the mother and the daughter, making the individuals and the whole family system unhappy and dysfunctional. Interpersonally harmful catharsis such as altercation and acting out seem to provide only momentary relief for emotional distress; also, it is not without regret, shame, and guilt. Mrs. Sim said, "I have just spoken ill of my daughter. However, I loosened and unknotted my mind *[maum ul pun da]*; that way, I feel a little cool and better inside."

INABILITY TO FORGIVE A GRANDCHILD

Mrs. Woo is a seventy-six-year-old widow with a middle-school education, who came to the United States in 1979. She told of her life experiences:

> There is nothing to be pleased about. I am just waiting for the day I die. I am close to eighty years old. I think I have been living too long. I'd like to die while I am still able to move my hands and feet. There were many friends of mine who died recently. When I lived with my eldest son's family, I was not lonely because I was mingling with my grandchildren. When I live alone, I feel lonely and sad. I try to spend time with my friends in my apartment. Against my children's wishes I moved out. This is the reason they do not support me, so I live rather poorly. I live very thriftily.
>
> I came to America by my eldest son's invitation because I really wanted to see him after a long separation. Living in America has been lonelier than when I was living in Korea. I feel at a loss because I cannot even communicate with my own children.

My ten-year-old youngest grandson's betrayal of me stays with me for a long time. He literally could not survive without me. I started to raise him as soon as he was born. Suddenly he changed his attitude altogether after I came back from a short visit to Los Angeles, and it made me very sad. Due to his betrayal, I felt the most painful despair to the degree that the sky and the earth became one [I was beside myself]. I was angry, sad, and lonely. I wanted to die because it was not fair. I cried every day for several months. I really like children and my love for my grandson was extraordinary. But after the incident, I decided that I would never love my grandchildren again, but would live only for my own life from now on. I resolved the distress all by myself since it was an embarrassing story to tell to others. But I have never forgotten that experience.

Because of the boiling heat inside me, my heart ailment got worse. Emotional turmoil and heart illness go hand in hand. My heart illness was most severe when my grandson betrayed me. I suffered from *hwabyung* at the time when my daughter-in-law said something agonizing to me, which was nailed on my chest. Then my heart illness got worse again. I felt like I was dying because my heart beat too fast.

Because of my grandson's betrayal, I moved out to where I live now. I thought that when my grandson did not like me, why should I bother to continue to live with him? However, he changed a lot recently. When I visit him, he even greets me. Recently I feel much better. Now I live alone so that there is no one to trigger *hwabyung* or heart illness in me. My family and friends are careful not to aggravate my condition.

Mrs. Woo sounds as though she lives on thin emotional ice, with a delicate balance and regulation for harmony within herself and persons in her circle. The Korean grandmother's emotion, mind, and soul could be injured by the perceived cold or indifferent attitude of the grandchild and his family, enough to cause her heart ailment. Mrs. Woo may have felt that her grandson should ask her pardon for his ingratitude for her true love and care. This kind of existential, psychological, and spiritual distress may cause physical pain. Her grandson might have felt the same way when his grandmother left for Los Angeles, probably without giving him any guidance. That might have been their first separation. That may have been why he exhibited the unexpected behaviors that his grandmother observed and felt. The situational anxiety may have made him numb and indifferent. I wonder if his grandmother and parents understood the likelihood of separation anxiety at his tender age. I am not sure whether she tried to understand her grandson's developmental feelings of abandonment before feeling her own betrayal and rejection.

What the grandson thinks of her or how he behaves toward her are very important generally to grandparents, because it tells them how they are valued and respected by the younger generation. According to Korean traditional family values, the grandmother serves as a nurturing surrogate for grandsons, the future patriarchs, and wants to contribute to perpetuating the lineage. If grandchildren value grandparents, then their adult children also value them, as the children's position is increasingly important in the family. If Mrs. Woo felt that her grandson liked her, she might not have moved out, because it would have given her a feeling of achievement, contribution, self-esteem, respect, and a sense of belonging. She must have felt that she wasted her lifelong investment.

Mrs. Woo might have felt that the young lord of the household did not accept her where she had served for her entire life. She feels she is an outsider in her own son's home in the nuclear family. She becomes even more inner-directed (Riesman, 1969) in adapting to the inevitable change in family values from collectivism to individualism. She could legitimately have been a matriarch in her household. She is longing for family togetherness and she seems to care about the role of matriarch in a traditional Korean family. Currently she enjoys her carefree, independent, tranquil life by herself, although she longs for closeness with her family.

Mrs. Woo might have been vulnerable because of her stressful immigration and fatigue from her travel to Los Angeles, and not able to accept her lonesome and estranged grandson right after their first sudden separation from each other since he was born. It must have been equally stressful for her grandson, causing his initial behavior to be awkward, regressed, somewhat indifferent, and even hostile to his grandmother. If only Mrs. Woo could have been strong enough to accept her grandson, with grandmotherly understanding, love, and care. However, she was not able to do so because she herself was shocked and preoccupied with regaining her own integrity, which was on the verge of a breakdown. It should be recognized that the grandmother's position in the nuclear family has become sensitive and vulnerable.

Mrs. Woo equates *hwabyung* with heart illness. Sometimes she presents heart illness as one of the phenomena of *hwabyung,* originating from distressed nerves because of disharmonious interpersonal relationships and misunderstandings. This seems to be a classic example of semantic networks of holism, as Good (1977) demonstrated about two decades ago.

Chapter 6

Family Life

This chapter presents stories of the conflicts, problems, and coping strategies related to parents' continued adherence to Korean family structure, social values, and styles while children have broken with tradition.

A COUPLE LIVING SEPARATELY FOR THE CHILDREN'S SAKE

Eighty-one-year-old college-educated Mr. Ro came to America in 1980, where he had lived for ten years at the time of our interview. He taught and later he was in business. He was married and had three sons and five daughters. He has "sugar urine disease" (diabetes) and gives himself a daily insulin injection.

> I lived comfortably in Korea because we didn't have to worry about putting food on the table at mealtimes. We had a business. We did not envy others because we had enough for an upper-class life. During the Japanese occupation I went to school. Our parents enjoyed raising us and appreciating us, and we distinguished ourselves in society. We supported our parents and raised our young children. During the Korean War, many horrible, tragic things happened, such as abandoning children during the escape from the war, killing people by dropping them into deep wells, shooting people with guns, etc. The communists killed my brother and his body could not even be found.
>
> The individualism in America is something different from the collectivism in Korea. An individual goes out to live only

for his own life. My son lets me use a small room in his house. I need to make myself emotionally and physically comfortable. There is no facility even if I want to exercise. Older Korean adults do not fit into American society. They have no place in America and they are not needed in America. They have language and transportation problems. I cannot expect my children to help me because they are busy with their work. My children brought me here. They told me a lie that America is a "paradise." My children made their mother a kitchen maid and their father was a useless man to them. Their mother was also expected to take care of the grandchildren and she is homebound. Men can go out with their friends. Our children feed my wife and me. I receive 160 dollars a month. I buy cigarettes and then there isn't much money left.

In America, you cannot see a physician right away. You have to make an appointment. Usually you have to wait at least two to three days. That is hard. Can an old person work? What can an old person do? There is nothing to feel good about. I cannot possibly describe the loneliness I am experiencing because it is very severe. I don't even need to talk about that. I am lonely day and night, perhaps because I do not have any hobbies to provide solace. Also, I cannot speak English, I can't go anywhere, so I just stay at home. Old people are useless. I am always lonely. It does not apply to me that sometimes I'm lonely and sometimes I'm not. If one understands the lonely situation, it is all right, but if not, one has regrets: Why did I come to America? I go to church and ask God to relieve my loneliness.

Here in America, in order to eat, everybody has to work and participate. It is good that the American social system was made so that everybody can eat whether you are white, black, or yellow.

When my parents passed away in 1977, I was very sad. I miss my parents who are no longer in this world and cannot come back. My vital energy was blocked when the sky tumbled down after my parents' deaths. My father is the sky and my mother is the earth. When the sky and the earth were tumbling down, my vital energy was blocked. However, when time passed, I forgot the grief.

> The pattern of depression is different from person to person. Depression depends on one's own cultivation of the whole self. Depression is not necessary. It is best to live optimistically. Depression is not an illness but a temporary symptom. It really does not matter whether I am depressed or not. I just wait for the day when I will die. I have been giving insulin injections to myself for twenty years. That is why I don't have other complications. I don't know how long I will live. What is certain is that I am alive now.

Mr. Ro talked about his experience with extended family living in terms of filial piety. He expressed his great sorrow in terms of lost vital energy upon his parents' deaths. His parents' existence was a vital force for his own spiritual life. Mr. Ro felt that his whole world was apocalyptic at his parents' deaths because his parents meant his whole world to him as the symbol and meaning of life. What he was feeling toward his parents was filial piety, mutual caring, and respect. He probably was comparing and contrasting his feelings toward his parents and toward his perception of his children's treatment of him and his wife. Mr. Ro might have supported his parents in the best room he had, probably the master bedroom, not a tiny room like the one given to him by his son's family. Mr. Ro himself might have lived and slept in the living room or kitchen if his parents were alive and he lived in a small apartment.

He expressed his feelings in terms of the sky and the earth falling apart. This traditional, cosmological expression is used in extreme, chaotic situations or when there is a catastrophic perception that one's main support system is failing. He was beside himself. Even though he is over eighty, he still has great respect and longing for his parents. He learned that the priority in an extended family is caring for elderly parents. He might have expected the same filial piety and care from his children that he gave to and received from his parents.

Mr. Ro concluded that he is neglected by the younger generation due to their busy lives; he feels useless and unwanted by society; and his wife is forced to do traditionally unappreciated labor for their children. He barely survives financially. He also found the appointment process for medical visits cumbersome compared to the walk-in clinics or drugstores in Korea. A pharmacist in Korea can prescribe or sell almost any medicine to people who walk in. He is disappointed with his lifestyle in America.

He believes that life should consist of more than eating, sleeping, and passing time meaninglessly. He wants to exert himself positively, but so far, he finds that his limitations in human resources, English, and mobility hinder him from doing so. He waits for death with the thought that it is almost time for him to go to the other world. There is a saying in Korea, "It is rare for a person to live to be seventy years old," while Mr. Ro is over eighty.

Mr. Ro defines death as a natural phenomenon that inevitably comes whether one likes it or not and that hopefully ends a meaningless and burdensome life. This is also the case for other elderly informants who feel they lead meaningless lives and feel that they are burdensome to themselves, their children, and others. Although they are not particularly unhappy, some elderly Koreans feel that they are ready to leave this world as part of the natural cycle. Mr. Ro ultimately finds peace with God.

Mr. Ro keeps his emotional equanimity, although he sounds unhappy. He is able to vent his feelings with an understanding of his reality. He does not see depression as an illness but as something one can control with willpower and self-control. In 1998 I tried to call to talk with him about his recent developments. His wife informed me that he had passed away. He was diagnosed with lung cancer and cataracts. About three years before his death, they had had a diamond jubilee for their sixtieth wedding anniversary. In America, Mr. and Mrs. Ro lived in separate homes. Although Mr. Ro was terribly lonely every day, he lived with their eldest son while Mrs. Ro lived with their youngest son in order to look after their grandchildren.

There is a Korean saying: "When an aristocrat is drowning, he would not swim like a dog." It may make him lose face. It is better to die with dignity. One has to live for harmony, honor, and respect, doing good for others. Apparently Mr. and Mrs. Ro wanted to live together but declined to for their children's sake. Mrs. Ro stayed where she could take care of her grandchildren. Mr. and Mrs. Ro and their adult children may have believed that elderly people do not need to live together. Mr. Ro visited Mrs. Ro sometimes. When

Mr. Ro was visiting Mrs. Ro for the last time, he stayed overnight and then went back to his eldest son. Although Mrs. Ro asked him to stay a little longer, he went back after telling her that there was no special reason for him to stay longer. Probably, intuitively, they wanted to spend more time together for the last time. But, because of the rest of his family and "the eyes of others" according to Confucian tradition, he might have felt that he should go back to his eldest son's place to finalize his worldly affairs. He probably did not want to disturb their children to accommodate him. A man who does not behave thoughtfully by considering others as a gentleman may be ridiculed in his old age. His daughters-in-law might whisper, "What is going on?" while his sons smile as they look at their parents. Mr. Ro was probably a Confucian aristocrat who would not allow that to happen in his family. He would not even think about breaking a routine without proper reasons. He readily maintained decorum, etiquette, dignity, and respect for others and self out of a lifelong self-cultivated discipline and judgment, following the Confucian way of life. It is oriented intellectually, logically, rationally, and ritually rather than emotionally.

Also, he probably had a premonition of his imminent death. After he returned to his home, he called his wife to let her know that he had arrived safely. That was the last interaction between them. Two hours later, Mrs. Ro heard the news that her husband had passed away. Dying with dignity and respect for the harmony and order of family and society is very important for Mr. Ro's last rite. Mrs. Ro regrets that she could not stay with her husband in his final hour in this world. She said, "Others said that that was good because he was able to go easily and quickly, but for me, I wish I had been able to be with him and take care of him even a little." They were longing for each other in their hearts even in old age.

A SON WHO OBEYS HIS WIFE'S COMMAND

Mrs. So, a seventy-eight-year-old widow, is a Christian with a middle-school education. She has been living in a subsidized senior citizen apartment for thirteen years in the United States. She has one son and one daughter.

I heard that my husband passed away while he was studying in France. But I didn't witness his death, so I have been waiting for him for about fifty years. But time is running out. It is soon time for me to die. I am old. My family, my relatives, and my friends have been telling me that I should be grateful because I have children from him at least. During the Korean War, I had hardships. We were very hungry.

I was asked to come to the United States to care for my grandchildren. I had missed my son very much, so I came right away. Then I really wanted to go back to Korea because I was disappointed in living with my son and daughter-in-law in America. I was sad, but I couldn't go back because I sold everything or brought it here and gave it to my son's family. My son was a devoted son in Korea, but he only cares for his wife in America. It is the way it should be, but it is too hard and foreign for me to understand. First of all, in Korea, a woman does everything for a man. But here in America, my son does whatever his wife orders him to do. It was a great disappointment, especially since my son is the only son in our three generations. I was so careful in what I said, how I said it, and how I behaved when I lived with my daughter-in-law, that I felt uncomfortable. That's why I left them to live alone in this senior apartment.

I am lonely, uncomfortable, and troubled as I get old and my friends die one by one. Only one of them is left. If one lives with one's spouse, he or she is not lonely. At the beginning, living all by myself was good, as if I found new freedom. We Korean folks gathered together and cooked and shared, but these days I have to do everything by myself. It is hard even to eat and be alive. In the past I was able to read the Bible; now I cannot do that because my vision went bad. When I am sick, I have to call my son. It has been very pleasant to live in this senior apartment, but there is no one to take care of me when I am ill. I had a mild stomach ulcer and a gallbladder inflammation because I used to worry a lot. I have been lonely for twenty years, ever since I came to America.

In Korea I sewed clothes for others. I worried a lot until my customer tried on what I sewed and went home satisfied. In

> America, it was fun at the beginning, although it was like living in a prison. Once a month we had meetings with friends for *ge* [a fund collected among trusted friends]. I learned Korean dancing at that time. I didn't mix with people well at the beginning like *quer da non bori jaru* [a person with an unsociable personality]. Later on, I was able to mix really well. We also met for occasions like a grandchild's one-hundred-day-old celebration, birthdays, etc. We ended up meeting three or four times a day sometimes. My son didn't like me to have so many frequent meetings, so I quit and started to go to the Korean church.

It was very hard for Mrs. So to accept the changes in the traditional Korean hierarchy. She believed in male dominance and female submission. But her son's marriage seemed to be the opposite way, according to her observation. She couldn't accept and tolerate that and she had to move out. To Mrs. So, her son was the most precious person in the whole world. She looked up to him and listened to him very carefully. If he did not approve of her behavior in the slightest, she discontinued it although it might be something she enjoyed and something perfectly legitimate. Mrs. So did not want her son to be dominated by his wife in any way. In Korean society, the only son or the eldest son is very respected and treated with utmost care. This is a typical source of conflict between mother-in-law and daughter-in-law.

Also, Mrs. So is sad about her lonely life and possible health problems in the future, although she enjoys her everyday life when she is with friends and when she goes to church. The origin of her sadness might be the difficulty of depending on her son. She stated, "Depression should be treated by one's own mind and will, but not by medication."

SHAME AND GUILT EXPERIENCES BECAUSE OF DEATHS IN THE FAMILY

Mrs. Hahn is a sixty-two-year-old Christian widow with a middle-school education. She was born in an aristocratic family and married into one as well.

I get angry [fire] and irritable easily. I don't respond kindly to my daughter when she comes home late because she doesn't let me know in advance why she is late. All I live for is my daughter. I worry to death about her when I don't know where she is. I get frustrated with the thought: "Even my child doesn't understand my concerns." I say, "Kill me, kill me," because the distress and worry ruin my health. We fight so often that my daughter is not gentle with me, and then I have regrets. I have to be patient but it is difficult for me to be patient. Now I feel cool inside of me because I have released everything accumulated in my body talking to you.

I came to America to see my pitiful daughter, who has lived alone since she became a widow about ten years ago. My son-in-law died of a heart attack suddenly. I cook and clean her house while she works. In America, I feel helpless because I can't communicate or go anywhere by myself.

My husband was killed during the Korean War when I was young, so I have lived with pain all my life. I realized that I lost all my family members who could support me. I was so ashamed of myself at their deaths that I couldn't go out for a long time. When my husband was killed, I couldn't go around with my head high. At my son-in-law's death, I felt dishonored and disgraced. When I was asked to go on a sightseeing trip to a famous mountain in Korea, I decided not to go because I was ashamed. But my daughter asked me to go and I set out. However, I felt as though people pointed their fingers at me because I was so ashamed of myself about his death. I thought I should be the one who should have died, not him.

My body aches. I think it is related to sadness and depression. I became a widow and so did my daughter. Alas, my daughter's fate is so pitiful. I live by overcoming loneliness and shame with my faith. Also, I am able to live because there are others who live in worse conditions than I do. I work hard to forget my misery.

Although she was not directly responsible, Mrs. Hahn may have felt ashamed, dishonored, and disgraced because she believed that her husband and son-in-law's untimely deaths were her fault, which was the result of her unlucky, cosmological fate according to her belief system. She seems to take moral and ethical responsibility. She feels she is not virtuous enough to deserve a happy family. She probably relates this to her karma. She may believe that she deserves these unlucky events because of evil behaviors committed in her previous life. Others may think that she was an evil person who causes evil things. She added Korean sayings about widows: "She is a bitch who ate up her husband" and "A widow makes up and dresses up for *param pium*" (having affairs with other men). If family members die, other family members (usually a wife, mother, or daughter-in-law) are blamed. Often self-blame is more severe than accusations from others. Mrs. Hahn felt as though she had been accused and had low self-esteem.

Mrs. Hahn believes that she has *hwabyung* because of the situation related to the family deaths and her current conflictual relationship with her daughter. She said: "You can't cure *hwabyung* with medicine or even traditional Korean medicine. You have to overcome it with your will. If not, it will develop into insanity or a stroke." Mrs. Hahn is familiar with the mental resolution of distress. She says that emotional distresses such as anger dwell in the body. She explains the psychodynamics between herself and her daughter in terms of a chain reaction. If only one would care for the other, the other person would also care for the first person in return, which is a Korean proverb: *"O nun chong i it ser ya ga nun chong do it da."* Ultimately, Mrs. Hahn is worried that she will lose her daughter as well because of her experience of repeated losses of close family members.

Chapter 7

Women's Lives: Has Marriage Been Bitter, Salty, or Hot?

Stories related to disharmonious marital and family relationships as perceived by women are presented in this chapter. Women's difficult and tragic as well as light moments are revealed in these stories. Their constructed and deconstructed illnesses are presented in context.

ENJOYING PEACE: FORGIVING THE UNFORGIVABLE THROUGH GOD'S GRACE

Mrs. Bang, a seventy-three-year-old widow with a high school education, has lived in the United States for eighteen years. At first she stayed with her daughter, but now she lives alone in an apartment. She has three children: one son is a professor, and the other son and the daughter have businesses.

> In my old age I am thankful to my children for living comfortably like this. I was able to come here with their support. When I am healthy, I do not have worries. I like my apartment. I live comfortably without even feeling it is cold or hot because of the good heating and cooling system. Transportation is convenient. I study English twice a week at the Korean elderly association. I am very thankful.
>
> Sometimes it is troublesome because I cannot speak English. I asked the people at the Korean community service

center to help me apply for financial assistance and medical aid because my children did not have time during the week. My daughter invited me to take care of her children because she was studying. I like to live alone quietly because of the generation gap. During the week I look after my grandchildren at my daughter's and during the weekend, I return to my apartment and spend time quietly with my friends.

I have not felt lonely. Loneliness seems to have something to do with one's personality. Besides, I was too busy for loneliness. One has to develop hobbies. On Sundays I go to church and listen to a good sermon so that I cannot be lonely.

In Korea I devoted my time to raising my children. My hobby was growing flowers. My husband established an art school. But, during the Korean War, we had a very hard time just feeding and clothing ourselves. We were fortunate just to be alive.

I experienced depression and sadness when my daughter died a year ago from cancer. I neither wanted to go anywhere nor ride in a car. My health deteriorated. I had no appetite and my eyesight was dim. I was that way because my mind, emotion, and soul were shocked because of my daughter's death. I have not gone to my daughter's grave because I do not want to experience the shock again.

I was practically out of my mind. I did not know whether it was day or night. I felt that I was bewitched by something. I did not want to hear what others said and I did not want to see the people who were talking to me. I was depressed and I talked much less than usual. I became passive and not interested in anything. My body became weak because I worried too much and was thinking too much about what to do and how to do it day by day. My mind must have been in a strange state. My head felt numb and my behavior was dull and slow. I felt something hard in my stomach and in my throat. I was crying softly and uncontrollably when I was breathing. I had palpitations and hypertension.

I was feeling sad and depressed enough not to want to live any longer. I did not have any thoughts. Sometimes I felt that my head was empty. I blamed God for letting death happen to my daughter and making me unable to think and do anything. I did not know what God's will was at that time. At last, I thought that God must have taken my daughter for his holy purpose and I was able to accept my daughter's death with better understanding. I was comforted when I knew that she went to God's wonderful heavenly realm. I began to understand other people who have experienced this same agony and I could sympathize with them.

What I told you about is depression and its symptoms. Every day I think about my daughter and I feel that my grandchildren from my daughter are to be pitied. At the beginning, the sadness and depression were very severe but, recently, it is better since time has passed. A classmate of my daughter visited her while she was sick. My daughter's church members kindly paid $1,500 toward her hospital expenses. My friends, who are like my real sisters, pray for me and give me solace.

I try not to be sad and depressed by reading the Bible, praying, and singing hymns in my bed at night. I listen to classical music and take walks. I concentrate on doing something so that I can occupy myself instead of being depressed. You have to overcome sadness and depression by yourself. If I do what I like, it helps how I feel and my health. My hobby might mean nothing to others, but it means a great deal to me. I like to decorate where I live. I try to forget and not to worry but to live joyously. Recently I found that I enjoy taking care of others because I have been through so much in my hard life.

For twenty-three years I suffered from *shingyungguamin* [similar to *shingyungshayak*] when my husband did not come home, did not take care of his family, for *param pium* [having affairs with other women], and again when he died.

However, *shingyungguamin* refers more to worrying and the problem-solving process than physical interference. It seems to be limited more to mental and cognitive distress than the physical aspect, while *shingyungshayak* is the involvement of mental as well as physical weakness due to *shingyungguamin*. Thus, *shingyungshayak* is the end product of *shingyungguamin*. *Shingyungguamin* and *hwabyung* are the same thing.

During the Japanese occupation my husband passed the Highest Civil Service Examination, which is recognized as the highest honor and privilege. He had money and he took bar girls to the mountains and hills for fun. The father of our children did not care for them, so that I had to take most of the responsibility for them. I worried also about our children's education. When we were living in Manchuria, and he did not come home for three or four days in a row because of *param pium,* I worried that he might have been attacked by bandits. We talked about writing a divorce paper about twenty times a month. I felt pressure on my chest and had feelings of suffocation. He made me worried and angry. When I talked to my friends about my marital problems, they said it was all right to divorce. Talking with friends helped me to put out the "fire" inside of me. They agreed with my idea of divorce. However, my birth family insisted that I had to become a ghost in my husband's family by living there until my death because they believe that I can be married only once in my lifetime. Divorce or separation is not allowed at all. Since I could not go to my birthplace, I agonized all alone. My husband had several additional mistresses and I had to stay home doing everything by myself.

It was so painful, as if my chest was exploding. I could not say what I wanted and I had to absorb the feelings all by myself. I could not digest what I ate and, naturally, it became an illness. My liver and intestines went bad. I could not breathe while I slept. In my case, it was worse during menopause. I felt something obstructed in my chest and I could not help sighing. When I could not breathe, I was fearful of dying suddenly. I learned finger pressure and therapeutic breathing methods and I practiced them on myself. I received tonic injections for about two months.

My husband had a stroke in his old age. I cared for him while he was having urinary and fecal incontinence. For three years, I washed him several times a day as well as changed his diapers soaked with urine and stool. I had more sympathy for him than anger. I said "You poor thing" to my husband in my mind. I gave him all the best nursing care I could give. With all

> my unfortunate experiences, everybody thought that I would die before my husband.
>
> When I became emotional, I turned on magnificent classical music and cried. There was something I could not yet decipher in my mind, emotion, and soul even with music. It was resolved and I was healed when I had a laying-on-of-hands ceremony in church. I think about things optimistically. I live actively. I resolve conflicts by talking things over with my friends. One can overcome anything if one believes in Jesus. My God healed me of the illnesses. I work harder in my church and I am connected with more friends through my faith in God. I feel wonderful because I talked to you about my personal life. I thank you very much.

Mrs. Bang calmly reminisced about her life in relation to her illnesses. She related her daughter's untimely death to her depression, and her husband's extramarital affairs and his death to her *shingyungguamin*. At some point, she was diagnosed with major depression using DSM-III. Mrs. Bang used the terms depression, *hwabyung,* and *shingyungshayak* interchangeably. She has understanding and supportive children who are successful, and she was doing well until her daughter's recent death. She described herself as having chaotic experiences that are out of order in the cosmological, mental, physical, psychic, and spiritual realms.

She had friends who shared similar values and supported her. She appreciates her own endurance and perseverance in maintaining her marital responsibilities all the way to her husband's final days, and still remembers her husband with compassion. When she lived in Manchuria, her whole family life was at stake in an unsettling, risky place and time. It might have been very difficult for her to take responsibility during her husband's long absence, as documented in a story about her cohort (Lee, 1996).

Actually, she wanted to divorce her husband, but her family and society did not allow it. She had conflicts between her desire for divorce and her parents' advice based on traditional values. As her mental health condition worsened, so did her physical condition.

She was able to forgive her husband and, in return, she received peace of mind. She enjoys her life after her difficulties, feeling that it was worthwhile on the whole. Romantic love is not always necessary in the Korean marriage. In Korean society, she, her children, her husband's family, and her family might have suffered from guilt and shame if she chose divorce or separation from her husband. Mrs. Bang was a typical *jogwanggichur* (first formal wife).

She described the phenomenon of her illness and how she managed it, partially with various natural nonmedical self-care strategies such as classical music, serious work with concentration, changing negative thoughts into positive ones, alternative cognitive and emotional thinking, and open friendships. At first, she was ambivalent toward God because of her misfortunes. However, she confessed that God ultimately unknotted her *han* that she couldn't resolve alone and brought her meaningful life. Her recovery would not have been complete without religious awakening, reconciliation, and atonement.

She attributed her satisfactory living conditions, such as the subsidized apartment that she enjoys, to her children and the government. Improved financial conditions strengthen family relationships. Mrs. Bang also uses other support systems as much as she can. The help from her confidants has been very efficacious. Although she did not elaborate about her relationships with her children, she suggested that there were intergenerational conflicts and tried to avoid them by living alone.

Mrs. Bang emphasized that she is able to enjoy peace because she learned a great deal about herself in relation to others through suffering from *hwabyung,* which seems to have a therapeutic role as well as being a sickness.

CONTINUED SUFFERING AFTER MANY LOSSES

Mrs. Park is a sixty-eight-year-old widow with a tenth-grade education. She tells about her *han:*

> My father passed away when I was three, and my mother when I was twelve. I married at seventeen and was widowed at thirty-two. I lost four sons and one daughter. They all died; rather, I killed them.
>
> My daughter invited me to America in 1980 and I have lived here for ten years. My first year I lived with my daughter and

son-in-law and I felt I was living in a prison. My relationship with my son-in-law was not good. He interfered with my life. It was very uncomfortable for me to live with him in my daughter's house. One day I had decided that I would not go back to my daughter's family. I wandered around here and there to my friends' places and others' houses and worked for them in order to survive for about four years. I moved out here in this apartment five years ago.

I just hope to die. What is the use of living? An old person like me! Lonely! Sad! And I cannot go out! I do not have "feet" [a car] to move around and do things. My daughter works, so she cannot visit me frequently. Finally I learned to ride the bus.

It is unbelievable that I am still alive instead of being dead. There is nobody who is as lonely as I am. I have been distressed and lonely. I am full of *han* and pessimism. My husband passed away in his youth. I have lived alone for thirty years. One of my sons died at the time of his college entrance examination. I fainted at his cremation. I must have committed many sins in my previous life. I ached all over due to *shingyungtong* [nerve pains]. My heart was palpitating, my eyes were red, and my head was hurting around that time.

How wonderful it was to live in Korea. I could go anywhere I liked and I could speak the language. However, even in Korea, I only lived because I couldn't die. It was a difficult life. There is no one who had hardships as I did in America. I can't speak although I have a mouth and I cannot go where I want to go even though I have feet. My only wish is that I can be in good health and die in my sleep. Dying is not sad, but being ill and sick is sad. When I am ill, there is no way to help myself. If I could live with someone as a couple, I would be fine. I have no other wishes.

I have been sad and depressed every day for more than thirty years. I curse my past. I am sad and lonely. My real life is all over already. The life I have now is empty and vain. I don't want to think about anything anymore. I have finished living all my endowed life. There are no particular reasons for my sadness and depression. I am just making myself sad and depressed. I just make myself miserable. There is nothing else I can do for myself. My *shingyung* [mind, soul, and emotions] will be injured and shocked. I cannot even talk to trees, stones, or Buddha. When a person has severe sadness and depression, *shingyung* will come out of the body and the person will become insane. The person will become a mental patient and eventually will die.

Three years after my husband passed away, my son died. At that time, I could not see anything and I could not figure out anything. I was not afraid of anything, even death. I didn't care about anything. I could not sleep even at four o'clock in the morning. I live only because my life is prolonged somehow. I cannot orget my dead children. *Bumo na nam pyon ie juk eu myon d'ang e mut go, jasik ie juk eu myon gasm e mut nun da.* ["People bury their parents and husband in the ground, but they bury their children in the bosom."] In order to forget I must die. There is no other way for me to forget.

I reminisce about my past because I am old. What sins did I commit in my previous life to make me so lonely now? Nobody understands my feelings and thoughts. I am too sad to see, to hear, or to shed tears. If one loses one's mind, emotion and soul, then he or she dies. But, my mind is clear. Whether man or woman, the person who lives alone is the most pitiful and miserable of all. A widow understands a widow's situation. Why did I pass my youth alone? Sometimes I think that I regret that I did not remarry. I cannot describe exactly my state of mind. I do not know even what and how I think anymore. Sometimes I wonder, if I had remarried, what would have happened. When I was busy raising my children, I didn't even think about remarriage. Now I regret that I did not remarry. If I die alone, who will know? Will my daughter know? Only ghosts will know. Sometimes I shout out to my children, "I spent all my youth to raise you, children!" I hope I can die just as I am. What I am longing for most is human compassion. I cannot comfort myself, although I tried to forget by drinking and listening to music. I learned to drink and smoke at the age of forty. I go out for fresh air at night when I feel I am suffocating from these miserable thoughts. I wander around to quell

> my unsettled mind, emotion, and soul. I dance in order just to cope. Actually, I love to have fun. I don't know how I have lived so long. Human life can be sustained and prolonged no matter how hard one's life has been. I know because I have experienced it myself.
>
> My troubled mind, emotion, and soul bring inner illness. My body parts become painful with *shingyungtong* [nerve pains]. My heart palpitates still faster. My eyes become red and painful. I get *hwabyung* like this when I am extremely lonely and when I am bothered with *shingyung*. I comfort myself by saying to myself, "You are suffering like this because you sinned a great deal in your previous life, so you deserve this suffering." I am somewhat better these days because I try not to be bothered with *shingyung* so much. When my mind, emotion and soul are troubled, diseases and illnesses come along. By the way, I don't care what others know about me.

Mrs. Park faced the deaths of her parents, husband, and children early in her life. She might not have had much opportunity to be loved and cared for by her family and to care for and love her parents, spouse, and children. She is begging for human warmth. She is full of grudges, guilt, remorse, shame, and self-pity. She said of her children, "Rather, I killed them." She did not literally kill them. But she expressed that she was taking moral responsibility for not being a perfect mother.

At times she said she is not certain about what she wants, feels, or thinks. She had conflicts with her son-in-law and wandered from this friend to that friend and even to strangers to make a bare living until she moved to subsidized housing. However, the move did not particularly seem to relieve her worrisome *shingyung*.

Probably she is preoccupied with her unhappy past and present loneliness, so that she is not able to appreciate her independence. She says that only by her own death will the agonizing memories and her present loneliness end.

She dwells on the negative side of her life (Beck, 1976). Therefore, she is not able to recognize the positive aspects of her life. She probably did her best to raise her children, but she blames herself and holds herself responsible for the tragedies in her family. She is never satisfied with her own goodwill and earnest efforts to care for others, no matter how hard she tries. She suffers from low self-esteem.

Mrs. Park has *han, hwabyung,* and *shingyungshayak*. Consequently she complained of bodily symptoms related to her emotional and spiritual distress. In essence, she is saying that she is biologically alive but was dead spiritually a long time ago. Koreans would say, "My inside is getting rotten" or "My inside is burning" when they are having emotional distress. I am wondering if this is an example of the relationship between sensation and mind (Shore, 1997: 44). The mind might be her negative thoughts and feelings, and sensation might be her perception of poor health. The point is that sensation could not exist without the involvement of the mind.

Mrs. Park was very open in expressing her thoughts and feelings, although sometimes she was not sure what she was feeling. She tried to convey her sense of loss and longing for an opportunity that she has not had so far because she was raising her children and conforming to the expectations of her family, society, and herself. She sounds bitter about her miserable fate. She may have expected filial piety from her children in her old age. The acculturation process, including living independently from her daughter, may have stressed Mrs. Park. Also, she is sad about her estrangement from her son-in-law.

Her helplessness and hopelessness intensify her misery. She did not mention an active spiritual practice of any kind or adequate self-care, although she seems to be familiar with Buddhism. She seems to say that she is too miserable to rely on any religious medium by saying, "I cannot even talk to trees, stones, or Buddha." Instead she drinks and smokes, although she knows that drinking and smoking are harmful to her health. Their value seems to outweigh the risk of cancer or disease in her mind. She has also tried meditation and diversion by walking in the fresh air.

Mrs. Park did not seem to derive any positive meaning from her hardships. But she is still searching for the true meaning of her life. She repeated several times, "What sins did I commit in my previous life to make me so lonely now?" She thinks of rebirth based on karma because she was taught about cosmological and cyclical phenomena in Buddhism. But she is not sure exactly what sins she has committed. She seems to be saying that if she has not committed sins, what other explanations are there? Perhaps after she answers the question, she may search for its meaning. She may be converted to Christianity and saved as her friends were, or she may seek the truth in Buddhism. Religion may be a way to strengthen her spiritually and give her a sense of well-being.

Some of her friends might evaluate her as a person of narrow personality and without a spiritual anchor. However, her situation, with an unusual lack of support from her children, other human kindness, and compassion could be significant.

Mrs. Park's emphatic and spontaneous narration of her life experiences, which she labels with Korean illness idioms related to depression, such as *han, hwabyung,* or *shingyungshayak,* has been her cultural healing process whether she recognized it or not. It was a cathartic outlet for her to reveal her accumulated thoughts and feelings with an active listener. I am hopeful that somehow she will resolve her agony by reviewing the events of her whole life and realizing the meaning of her long, painful loneliness and come to terms with it to bring change and peace to her soul. After all, she did her best, under the circumstances, for others and for herself.

ACHIEVING HEALING AFTER INJURY TO THE MIND, EMOTIONS, AND SOUL

Mrs. Cha is a sixty-five-year-old widow with a grade-school education who has been living in the United States for twelve years. She shared these experiences:

> Our son, from my second husband, invited my husband and me to America in 1979, and we lived with him for a year. Then we got our own apartment. I still feel like a guest in America. Material things, such as food, are better than in Korea. But I am always lonely here. About a year ago, my second husband passed away after our thirty-two-year marriage. So I feel very lonely in this apartment. I try not to bother my children if I can manage by myself. I try to overcome difficulties as much as I can, and I try to be patient.

She expressed an unsettled, homesick mood and a longing for family togetherness, care, and support:

> My life in old age is so-so. It is the same everywhere. Wherever you go, living in this world is all the same. When one gets old, one does not have much time to live. I do not speak to Americans because I do not know how to speak English. I cannot go anywhere I like because I do not know how to get there and I do not have a car. It troubles my mind.

These kinds of thoughts and the reality of life for the elderly have been addressed by most of the informants. She continued:

> My mind was seriously injured in my youth because I failed in my first marriage. I wanted to become a ghost in my first husband's family [faithful and loyal to her husband and his family until her death]. My husband started to *param pium* when I was pregnant for the first time, at the time of Korea's independence from Japan. My husband played with this woman and that woman even when he was a bachelor. I did not know that because it was an arranged marriage. Also, he was from a shaman's family, which usually makes people uncomfortable.

Shamans tend to be looked down on and they are avoided because of their reputation for possessing supernatural powers. People are afraid of being affected by their powers. People are reluctant to associate with them because if others know of that kind of connection, they are stigmatized. Mrs. Cha continued:

> What made me even more distressed, helpless, and hopeless was that my mother-in-law and my four sisters-in-law were defending and supporting my husband's extramarital life instead of reproaching him. I had two daughters. My mother-in-law hit my daughters. I tried to visit my daughters in their primary school, but they avoided me. After I left my first husband's house, almost by being chased away by my mother-in-law and sisters-in-law, one of my daughters disappeared.
>
> My mind, emotion, and soul are painful. I feel as though clouds have accumulated in my mind, emotions, and soul. I never have moments when I am happy. Basically, I neglected and dumped my daughter. Probably, I should have brought my

children with me at that time, but I did not do that because I did not have any means to raise them. It is still a painful memory. That is why my mind, emotion, and soul are painful still. A lot of times, I wanted to die and I tried to die because of my estranged daughter, my failed first marriage, and the death of my second husband. I have been depressed for forty years. The saddest time was when I was separated from my own child who was born from my body and soul. I tried to die together with my children, but it did not happen that way. When I reflect on it, I am sure that all those terrible things happened with God's will in Christianity to rescue me from my unhappy marriage in a shaman's house. A troubled mind, emotion, and soul cause depression and sadness. If I live with my children, I won't feel so lonely.

I married for the first time at the age of twenty-one and divorced at twenty-six, and lived alone for ten years. Then I met my second husband, who had two children already with his previous wife, a boy and a girl. It was very hard to raise the children whom I did not bear.

I suffer from indigestion, which is psychogenic. I comfort myself by thinking there are people who are worse off than I am. I want to hear from my daughter who has disappeared. I wish I could visit my hometown in Korea. I am very sad and depressed. When I think about my past, my eyes fill with tears. Also, I feel that my throat feels uncomfortably full with a lump when I am sad. I try to forget, and I do not usually reveal my sad past to others because I do not want to look sad and miserable.

In order to forget my sad situation, I read the Bible, sing hymns, and spend time with friends. Sometimes it is hard although I try to be content with myself. I go to pleasant places, laugh, and forget. However, it is just temporary. There is no permanent cure. Besides, I cannot go to places all the time. I have to find solace in my mind, emotions, and soul, and live day by day.

Depression and sadness are related to *shingyungshayak,* which causes indigestion. I gave up life's joy and happiness. What else is there for me? Nothing. Dying is the best for me. How can I overcome my troubles? Nobody knows my troubles.

> If other people could go inside of me and look, then they might understand me. There is no other way. I am experiencing agony when nobody is aware of it. I am ashamed of myself. What a nerve I have! I talked about my daughter whom I abandoned. I am guilty of that.

This narration reflects that the informant perceives herself as a victim of her husband, mother-in-law, and sisters-in-law at the time of her first marriage around 1945, at the end of World War II. She expressed grave shame and guilt from her alleged abandonment of her daughter, and suffered from it. Her self-blame is obvious, although Mrs. Cha's disadvantaged situation did not allow her to take her daughter with her and raise her; the husband's family has custody rights for children in Korea (Koh, 1983). It is very hard to raise a child alone, economically and socially. A stigma is attached to a child who has been raised by an abandoned single mother.

Mrs. Cha interpreted that she embodied the troubles of her life, and the embodied troubles afflict the mind, emotion, and soul. Mrs. Cha described *shingyungshayak* as a physical disease caused by emotional distress from disharmonious family relationships. All of this was experienced by Mrs. Cha before she became a Christian. She believes that a structural change or other changes could be visible, and they could be different from those of the average person. Her beliefs demonstrate her body-mind, cognitive, emotional image and reality. Her emotional injury is just like a bodily injury.

She was concerned enough to wish that someone, especially an intimate and significant person such as a confidant, would hear and understand her life experiences, so that she could be healed. She tried hard to explain exactly what happened in her life, what she thought of her life, what emotional conflicts she had, and how she did her best under the circumstances. However, losing her daughter injured her inside and out. She blames herself and takes that as her responsibility. She wants to hear someone say: "You did your best under the circumstances. Sometimes unfortunate things happen even though you try to do everything right. God takes care of what we cannot." Her unfinished task is to find her missing daughter—perhaps in Korea. That may be why she wishes to visit Korea, besides the homesickness that she feels.

When she was contacted five years after the original interview, she said she believed in God and was able to reconcile the agony and distress related to her past and is content with her present life. Her husband died from complications of diabetes. The only thing she is concerned about these days is what to do when she no longer can take care of herself. She is determined not to live with her children but might go to a nursing home in America or in Korea. She is not sure what to do. Although one of her daughters and a niece in Korea asked her to come and live with them, she does not think she would do that unless she could take a lot of money with her. Money might facilitate interpersonal relationships, and of course it helps in day-to-day living.

She has not yet really talked openly about how she will live if she loses her independence in America, and she doubts that she ever would have a chance to do that because it is such a delicate, taboo subject. She seems to secretly wish that whatever comes or happens, it will be taken care of somehow. Usually, neither elderly parents nor their children initiate planning about care arrangements or matters related to death. On the contrary, it is all set and understood between them by insight and intuition, through empathy and without actual talking (*yshim junshim*). Whether it is true or not, it seems to be taken care of somehow when it actually comes to that point. Planning might be better in terms of expediting the matter in a conventional sense, but in terms of dealing with a delicate and potentially risky intra- and interpersonal commitment, discussions tend to be avoided until absolutely necessary.

MATERIALLY POOR BUT FREE OF HWABYUNG *AND LIVING BY FAITH*

Mrs. Jin is a seventy-year-old widow with no formal education who has lived in the United States for ten years.

> My life in old age is a little tough because I don't have money. Money is the only problem I have. It is very difficult when we cannot pay the rent for our apartment. Sometimes I do housekeeping or baby-sitting to help my son pay the rent. We barely live with welfare and food stamps. My son has a job installing

siding, but a lot of times there are no siding jobs to do. My son is married but his wife has not come to the United States, so I live with my son. I applied for an apartment so that I can live there alone when my daughter-in-law comes here.

If I returned to Korea I would have to work in a rural area. I farmed and sold vegetables and fruit to keep us alive and I raised six sons and daughters. Grandfather (I mean my husband—I call him as my grandchildren do) broke his arm while plowing, but we could not take him to the hospital because the river was too swollen for us to cross the bridge due to heavy rain. So his right arm had to be amputated while he was young. This was an agonizing moment in my life. Grandfather just drank and did not work, saying, "I am disabled. How can I work?" So we sold our farm and paid our debts. We moved to another place and I started to work as a peddler with a basket full of goods on my head. Grandfather passed away at age sixty in Korea after he had prepared to come to America and all the documents for immigration had been filed. I could not even go to see him at his funeral. He could have been drowned in a heavy rain. I gave some money to a person who was on his way to Korea, and asked him to find out what happened to my husband. On this person's return to America, I was told that we were not informed about my husband's death by phone or letter because we might be startled and concerned about his death. I do not think I can work on a farm in Korea now although my family there asked me to return to Korea. If I cannot work on a farm, I have to guard our house. But I do not want to do that.

At the beginning of my immigrant life, I was lonely and frustrated in America. My daughter had suspicions about her husband, who was in the military. She even suspected me for something gone wrong with her or in her household. So I couldn't go to my daughter's place. According to rumor, she is separated from her husband and lives alone. When her condition becomes severe, she goes to the hospital and says that her mother sent her. I have a great deal of trouble with my daughter. I lived with my daughter for six months from the time I arrived in America and then she was suspicious of me, so I

> lived in someone else's house where I did baby-sitting and housekeeping. My biggest problem is the awkward relationship with my daughter. I wish my daughter would visit me. I cannot visit her because she does not like me to visit.
>
> My thirty-year-old son was killed in a car accident. He had left home in the morning and did not return although it was quite late in the evening. After ten o'clock, the hospital informed us that an accident had happened to my son. When I got there my son was already dead. It was too tragic. Empty feelings engulfed me. I was numbed. I thought of wanting to, at least, touch my son's cold hand. However, I was not allowed to touch his hands and I was not even allowed to go to the room where he was. I only could see him through a glass window. I was just shocked. I did not behave in any particular way though. I felt terrible and had helpless, empty feelings at that time.
>
> I look out through the window. When I feel stifled due to my son's death and my daughter's unhappiness, I smoke. I go to a Catholic church so that lately I do not feel so lonely. I am not particularly depressed. When I am fearful and feeling bad, I pray. When I am worried, it is best to depend on God and it gives me joy and makes me peaceful. I overcome the distress with prayer. Prayer is the only thing that works. I have never been hospitalized. I smoke and then I feel better. Family members and fellow churchgoers comforted me and prayed for me. I am just thankful for them. I am nothing really but they kindly helped me.

Mrs. Jin initially denied having a depressed mood but later admitted she did. She prays as a Catholic and did not develop *hwabyung*. Her self-care method is to faithfully pray and humbly accept support from others.

Her mixed reminiscences with regrets for painful situations and unfulfilled dreams are apparent. She enjoyed a brief sense of relief for having enough to eat and a roof over her head, but regretted not being able to educate her children and feels that her lack of education is the origin of her present poverty.

Mrs. Jin planned for her son to live in a nuclear family after her her daughter-in-law came from Korea. She is following a trend of changing role and function from the traditional dominance of the mother-in-law to that of the daughter-in-law (M. H. Kim, 1996).

Mrs. Jin expressed true sorrow over seeing the body of her dead son. She had to face a glass barrier, preventing her from bidding a final farewell by touching her son's hand. Korean parents would say: "Parents bury their child in their bosom when their child dies before they do."

Mrs. Jin has experienced the prevention and healing of depression through religious belief and faith. The support of their children is very important to elderly Koreans. However, Mrs. Jin's children were not in a position to support her. This informant, with a poor economic situation, is motivated to earn money in her own way. She regretted that she couldn't go to her husband's funeral. Perhaps she was not notified about her husband's death because they were estranged and had drifted away from each other, having lived so far away over many years. So, with awkward excuses, did someone in her family or other relatives in Korea decide not to send notice because of her advanced age and the difficult family and financial situations she was facing? Even devoted children and understanding relatives often do not let elderly parents know unpleasant news.

DEPRESSION: A PERSONAL EXPERIENCE

Mrs. Lee is a sixty-year-old widowed Christian who had volunteered to do prison work in Korea.

> I experienced sadness and depression. My eldest son died in a car accident. One of my daughters is still suffering from a mental illness, and my husband died suddenly of liver disease. I worried a great deal. My daughter has been in and out of mental hospitals. I feel that my husband could have lived a little longer if I had taken care of him well, because he had been healthy until he had the liver disease. My youngest son looked pitiful when he lost his father so suddenly.
>
> Still I feel sad and depressed, especially when the weather is cloudy or rainy and when the sun is about to set. I don't have

depression as an illness though; it is not severe. It is relatively mild. It didn't last a long time. It lasted for a few months. If it is prolonged, no one can live and he or she becomes a failure.

In Korean traditional medicine, depression is named *hwabyung*. Depression and *hwabyung* are similar to each other. I felt suffocated, as something seemed to be pushing up in my chest. I sighed rather often. I experienced it every day for several months. It is not so painful these days. When I am tired, I have a little angina. It is difficult for me to breathe because my chest hurts. Then it became heart disease. I recovered naturally as time passed.

It was mental pain and pain in my heart. I felt strange, that my mind was lonely and painful. I didn't want to do anything in the whole world and I didn't have any desire. I didn't want to speak with anyone. I didn't want to work and I didn't have any rules or routines in daily life. It was chaotic. I didn't feel that there was any hope for me. I walked alone endlessly. Silently, silently I thought as I looked up at the sky and trees. I walked where it was very tranquil and there was nobody.

I couldn't find anything interesting. When I am not busy, I am sad and depressed, so I keep myself busy to forget all the unpleasant matters by visiting and helping my youngest son. I comfort myself this way. Sooner or later everybody will be going back [death] to where he or she is from. I try to forget about the deaths of my son and husband, as I believe that they went to heaven and are living peacefully, and we can all meet again there one day. When my children were not around, I cried alone. I mean I wailed then. I felt I could breathe fresh cool air a little.

I tried to overcome my distress by myself and I wanted to stand firmly on my own feet. Some people helped me to laugh and some comforted me. My minister's wife tried to help my youngest son but it wasn't really helpful. People don't understand what one is going through until they experience what he or she is experiencing. I didn't talk about my family or our troubles to others. People can twist even good stories and they lose the original meaning when it gets around. Bad stories will

> get worse, I am afraid. For the first time, I feel something nice and cool inside of myself because I talked with you about everything I kept inside of me.

Mrs. Lee denied having depression as an illness but described it as a mood, although she was diagnosed as having major depression according to DIS-III criteria. There was a discrepancy even though the original DIS-III was modified according to Korean sociocultural and medical contexts. She tended to minimize her depressed condition. Perhaps she was being stoic because she was used to hardships. She appeared to equate depression and *hwabyung,* but the experience of "something pushing" (a lump) was described only in connection with *hwabyung*, not with depression.

Guilt feelings were provoked by her husband's sudden death because she felt that she did not provide the best possible care for him. She managed her dysphoric symptoms primarily by self-control. Everyone in her household suffers silently, all alone. However, Mrs. Lee seemed to feel that if the whole family understood their loss and cared for one another, the tragedies would affect all the family members less. Forgetting, through time, is used for natural healing. Talking about the painful experiences is discouraged because it is seen as a reminder of the unbearable pain of loss and tragedies. Talking about tragedy is like opening an already extremely painful wound with a sharp knife. She confessed that she was not sure whether the pain she was experiencing was physical, mental, or emotional. It could be thought of holistically. She was sure that her behavior was affected.

Although Koreans live closely in an extended family setting, the emotional climate is restrained. Each family member creates an emotional world according to his or her age, gender, hierarchical position, function, and role in the family structure, as in Mrs. Lee's case. Interestingly, Mrs. Lee mentioned that her minister's wife was not able to be empathic toward her emotional pains or to her son, although she tried to help. Mrs. Lee sounded disappointed, and she realized that people do not understand what others go through, even the wife of a clergyman. Mrs. Lee might be suggesting the value of a truly understanding and supportive person or professional help. Apparently, empathic active listening was helpful to Mrs. Lee, although the plain reminder of tragedy is discouraged among Koreans.

REGRET AND ANXIETY IN ANTICIPATION OF DEATH

Mrs. Yang is a seventy-nine-year-old widow with a college education. She has lived in America for ten years. She started by talking about her experiences with her husband.

> My husband was a high-ranking government official in Korea. When my husband suffered a stroke and became a hemiplegic, I felt that the sky and the earth were collapsing together [extremely shocked, chaotic, helpless, and hopeless]. I was beside myself. It gave me serious financial, emotional, and physical difficulties. My life was empty. I was very depressed.
>
> I didn't have any time for myself because I had to take care of my children and husband, who had the stroke due to hypertension. However, all my children went to the best universities and did well, and it made me happy and helped me overcome the hardships I was facing.
>
> I had severe arthritis and neuralgia. I had surgery after suffering a long time from it. Now it seems to be all right. I go swimming and to the sauna every other day. In my old age I am not afraid of dying. But I fear crossing over the boundary between life and death, and how I will die exactly. I don't know how people die really. I fear the unknown part of death. I wish I could die in my sleep without pain, without being aware of it, and without it taking a long time.
>
> Life is in vain. In my old age, I regret that I have lived an easy, worldly life. I had a great deal of fun. I loved to eat and travel. But now it seems useless and unworthy. I wish I had known a better way of living in my youth. I wish I had lived a worthy family and community life by sacrificing myself. I wish I had been more thoughtful, kind, and loving to my parents and husband. I have a great deal to do. I realize now that I want to live a worthwhile life from one moment to the

> next, so that I will not have any regrets. I want to enjoy life in a true sense but not for easy and pleasurable ways.
>
> Due to my language and transportation problems, I depend on my children, although I know that they are very busy. I try to learn English, but I just don't remember what I have learned. I appreciate the time and freedom that I have to do anything I want to do. I enjoy spending time with my friends. I still would like to travel a long distance.

Mrs. Yang concluded that she had a good life overall. She endured hardships for her husband and her children. Elderly Koreans value happiness related to family solidarity, their spouses, their children's educational status, high socioeconomic position, health, and material resources. She seems to have all these things, although there were significant difficult times in her life. Her children's excellent academic performances eased and lightened her heart and helped her to endure her hardships. Children's well-being, prosperity, and success are considered most important to parents, and children make sure that they are doing their best for their parents. However, while it would be almost unthinkable for most of the other informants, Mrs. Yang mentioned the importance of a sense of self as an independent individual separated from the family's well-being. Mrs. Yang was aware of the importance of leisure and actually took time to enjoy it, to the degree that she regretted indulging a little too much. This seems a little different from other informants. Probably it is because she, as a college graduate, is more educated than the other informants and she had financial resources from her husband. Still, she considers family matters as the highest priority. It seems that she regrets not having done enough for others in her community according to her standards.

Mrs. Yang specified her fear of death in terms of the phenomena and the process between life and death. I think she meant the moment of transformation from life to death, a moment she is afraid to experience. Mrs. Yang was able to talk about her fear of death candidly, which was a therapeutic catharsis.

According to Sister H. Suzuki's (1996) talk about her own momentary "experience of death" and other people's deaths, she concluded that it could be the most beautiful and spiritual event that one can experience.

Mrs. Yang did not mention Korean folk illnesses, although she recognized her depressed mood when her husband suddenly was disabled and she had to take on responsibility for the whole family. Perhaps she was able to overcome her hardships with available resources, her higher educational background, and support from her own children. She did not use Korean popular illnesses to explain her difficulties. Because she is more educated than most of the other informants, she prefers not to speak in terms of folk illnesses, or perhaps her hardships were not serious enough to cause depression or *hwabyung,* for example. Also, she is not used to experiencing Korean illnesses as a self-healing process.

"I LAUGH WHEN PEOPLE SAY THEY HAVE HWABYUNG"

Mrs. Yi is a seventy-eight-year-old widow with no formal education, who has lived in America for twenty years. Mrs. Yi cheerfully said:

> It's good to live in America. We are given money and an apartment to live in. If our children give us money, would they give it to us like that? I mean so generously, thoughtfully, and regularly? We can still live although we cannot speak English. In Korea, people don't look at your face but your clothes. That made me feel bad. They judge people based on how well one is dressed but not the person.
>
> I don't have depression. My husband brought in concubines to our house to live together and they bore six children. My friends told me that I was strange and I was an idiot because I was not angry in such circumstances. I laugh if people say they have *hwabyung* or *shingyungshayak* or depression because they don't know how to turn around their mind to positive directions. Also, they have to know that they are much better off than those people who are in worse conditions. If they can switch the negative thought, then they can forget the distress and they will relieve conflicts and they will be consoled and

happy. I don't keep grudges inside. I talk with friends. I sing hymns and songs in my mind and read the Bible. I forget unpleasant things.

Actually I enjoyed myself by visiting friends, etc. Still, I kept the formal wife's position because my husband's concubine took care of her children as well as my husband when he vomited after being drunk.

I heard through my brothers that my husband regretted treating me like that and he wanted me to come to him in Korea. But I didn't go. I knew his intention too well. He was living with another woman. I wrote to him before his death: "Don't be too hard on yourself. I have forgiven you. Live well in God's love." He wrote me back saying that he was sorry and he wanted me to come to him. My husband died six years ago. I went to Korea to attend his funeral ceremony. I feel very light in my mind. If I hadn't written to him to forgive him, I don't think I would be as peaceful as I am now.

I have nothing worthwhile left on earth although I have lived to an old age. I am not a learned person, so I have not written anything to mark my existence in this world. As I regret my unfulfilled life, I think of the people who are in a position worse than mine, and it helps me to console myself. My spirit becomes a little sad. I wish I could fly lightly and splendidly and shout loudly.

When I hear that someone died peacefully, easily, I say, "That is good," since I am old now. And I pray that I will die in my sleep comfortably, not giving others a hard time. I really don't worry about my death. I believe that I will be going to heaven. I prepared what I will be wearing when I go there. Because I believe in God, he will be taking care of me whatever situation I may be in.

Mrs. Yi's friends believe that Mrs. Yi behaves differently from what she thinks. In her circumstances, she had to be furious and jealous of her husband's concubines, according to her friends. She is supposed to have *hwabyung, shingyungshayak,* and *han.* However, Mrs. Yi denies it. According to her friend, she should take some kind of revenge on the concubines and even her husband, or some kind of defense to maintain sanity in her mind and faith in the institution of marriage. In Korea she is considered to have open-mindedness and self-cultivation. Some of her friends conjectured that she might have been born as a "man with a woman's mask" because it is believed that a man can have a generous mind but not a woman. Through several interviews, she explained that she did not do anything jealous or vengeful, as her friends expected, because of her upbringing in the Confucian tradition by her parents before her marriage. Humans should not be harmful or ugly to others. A woman should be virtuous. Another reason for maintaining her dignity and respect was that her mother-in-law was doing everything possible to rescue her marriage by begging or scolding her son or making Mrs. Yi pretty in her husband's presence. Still another reason for her relaxed attitude about her husband's extramarital affairs was that in a way she was proud of her husband because he was well-to-do and popular with women so that she was just pleased to be his legitimate wife.

In fact, her husband's marital betrayal hurt her deeply in her heart, although she suppressed her feelings and behaved as a cultivated, virtuous lady. That is why she may have said that she wished to fly and shout at the top of her lungs to get rid of the feelings of suffocation. She also said, "My husband transmitted all sorts of venereal diseases to me and I couldn't have more children, especially a son." Bearing a son is considered the most important duty and responsibility of a legitimate wife, but she couldn't continue to bear children after her husband had relationships with concubines. She verbally denied having *hwabyung* or *han* but her behavioral symptoms apparently indicate that she has been suffering from *hwabyung*. She, as her husband's first legitimate, legal wife, could not bear a son regardless of the reasons and, as a result, she is lacking or even disqualified from continuing to be the first wife. Therefore, she might have been expected to allow her husband's family to invite a concubine. In certain circumstances, in her situation, a thoughtful, legitimate wife makes arrangements to bring in a woman to bear a male heir, although Mrs. Yi did not mention it.

Her self-help strategy for seeking a contented life helped her live constructively. She repeated that she had to see a situation worse than hers so that she could be content.

When she looked back on her past she felt she didn't live a meaningful life for herself, others, or the community. She regretted that she didn't convert many people to Christianity when she was able to do so because she didn't realize its vital importance when she was young. Again, she could quickly be calmed by the thought that there are people worse off than she is. This way of thinking has become one of her cognitive coping strategies. She uses it in all situations and it appears to be efficacious for her.

I believe that Mrs. Yi suffered from *hwabyung* although she did not want to admit it. According to her explanatory model and semantic networks, her *hwabyung* journey healed her, brought her peace, and secured her a place in heaven.

Chapter 8

Men's Lives: "I Have to Cook and Do the Wash Although I Am a Man"

These stories relate the experiences of elderly Korean men in their former lives in Korea and their present lives in America. The meaning of their lives and scenes of vulnerability often without their wives or children are depicted.

A LONELY KOREAN GENTLEMAN

Mr. Moon talked openly about the common concerns and experiences of elderly Korean immigrants. Aspects of his day-to-day life included: his children, loneliness, health beliefs, death, financial matters, being elderly, life as an immigrant, marriage, living away from his children, religious opinion, becoming a U.S. citizen, widowerhood, life in America, depression, Korean folk illnesses, self-help, and so on.

Mr. Moon, eighty years old and college educated, had leadership positions in education, administration, and business in Korea. He has been concerned about his unhappy marriage and intergenerational family conflicts. He enjoys talking about his life. He told me that he is writing his autobiography and was wondering what to include and what to leave out because he is afraid that his first daughter-in-law and his daughter will be upset enough to tear up his book if he includes true stories about their unfilial behavior. He appreciates a conversation with someone who understands him, especially because it helps him to forget his loneliness.

Luckily I went to prestigious universities in Korea and Japan. I held a few high-ranking positions in Korea in the education and information field. I worked for the government as an administrator and did gold mine work afterward. My friends cheated me materially. I was good at leadership and public speeches. Huge crowds were very impressed with my speeches. I really worked hard and enjoyed my work at that time.

I have been living in America for twenty-one years. I came to America in 1975. I have three sons and three daughters. Upon my arrival in America I lived with my eldest son. I live alone now. I smoke. I could not learn English and driving due to my poor health, which is related to my stomach operation.

I was very unhappy with my marriage. My wife didn't even graduate from primary school and she acted like an idiot. She was insensitive and was not cooperative in my public life. She was stubborn, sticking to her old ways. When I was talking with other women, she was not even jealous of them or me. Yet she didn't want to divorce although I told her that I would give her everything I had. One day she stamped [the counterpart of signing in America] the divorce document under pressure from me, although she really didn't want to be divorced. Korean women of her age were not expected to divorce no matter how chaotic their marriages were. She knew that our children would not permit the divorce. After all, I didn't divorce for our children's sake and for moral reasons. My children didn't want me to divorce. If I were given the same situation again, I would definitely divorce because I sacrificed my whole life and it has not been worthwhile. By the way, my wife died a few years ago. During our marriage, we lived separately anyway.

My daughter invited me to come to America. My children are doing pretty well. Most of them have businesses except my youngest daughter, who had a car accident and has been receiving disability benefits. My second son gives her money sometimes to help her.

I helped my eldest son at his all-purpose store because it was boring for me to stay all day at home. I made sure that the goods and souvenirs for tourists were safe from thieves. I was elected president of an association for the elderly in the Korean community in Washington, but I resigned a month later because the members fought among themselves, abused public funds, and looked down on others.

I felt I was burdening my eldest son's family. When I lived with my son, I took care of my two grandchildren. I woke them up, bathed them, dressed them, fed them, and sent them to kindergarten and school while my son and daughter-in-law went to sell gifts to tourists from a wagon under a tent in Washington, DC. Also, I took the trash down from the third floor.

My health went bad after my stomach surgery. My daughter-in-law, who did not appreciate the baby-sitting and other work that I did, only reproached me, saying that I did not rear my grandchildren properly. My depressed mood is very severe because I have been depressed several times a day for a long time until now. I was most sad when my daughter-in-law said, "I don't know who but someone in this house has to move out."

Now that I live alone, my children do not visit or call me. I am most depressed when there is disharmony in my family, particularly with my children and daughter-in-law. I always feel depressed. This is depression. I feel utterly lonely when I return, all by myself, to my apartment from a visit to other places. It is worse because I live alone. I hope I can get a girlfriend.

After I had an altercation with my daughter-in-law, I felt sad and angry. As I told you already, I took care of my grandsons, but she did not appreciate that. Instead she reproached me for not taking care of them correctly. My daughter-in-law insinuated her wishes to me about moving out. One cold winter night I went to a bus stop to go to New York where my other children are. But I did not know which bus I should take. I waited and waited. I was very cold and started to cry. And I fainted and collapsed. Policemen came and so did an ambulance. My first daughter-in-law must have been aware of what happened at that time and apologized to me for her maltreatment toward me.

However, eventually I departed from my eldest son and my daughter-in-law, and went to my younger son and helped him with his flea market for three years including the hot summers and the cold winters. I regretted that I came to America. Finally

I moved out to live by myself. My children hardly ever call me or visit me. I go around by bus. My own children hate my eldest daughter-in-law because she did not treat me right. My children in New York and New Jersey hardly visit me. Their explanation for that is that they can visit only me but not my eldest daughter-in-law because they are not talking to each other. They are saying how can they visit only me and not her when they come to Washington.

I told you about my eldest daughter-in-law's unfriendly behavior to my second daughter-in-law. My daughter criticized me for repeatedly talking about useless matters. My daughter got married to an American. She invited our whole family to America. That is why she has become bossy with all of us. By the way, I like my American son-in-law very much. He is a good man. As soon as I heard what my daughter told me, I got really sad and angry, and I felt as though my heart got ruptured and I had to go to an emergency room. The Western medicine from the hospital did not work. So I am taking Korean traditional medicine and it is helping me. I told my daughter that when I die I will haunt her for three years and then I will take her with me. She gave me three hundred dollars at that time. I returned it to her right away.

I just got back from a trip to visit my children. My youngest son followed my advice to become a businessman. He has his own firm with many employees and earns one million dollars a year and built a huge house for his family with state-of-the-art technology near a beautiful park. Music comes out all over and doors open and close automatically. Everything is automatic, even the lawn sprinkler.

These days I cannot sleep because welfare benefits might be cut for non-U.S. citizens. Today I submitted an application for citizenship. I heard that if one has lived in the United States for more than fifteen years, someone else can answer the examination questions for U.S. citizenship in English for the non-English-speaking immigrants. A lot of people are having difficulty becoming citizens because of language problems. When no welfare benefits are available, older Korean immigrants should go back to their children, go back to Korea, or kill themselves. It would be very difficult to go back to their children, and matters will be very complicated in that case.

My health has not been good since my abdominal surgery was performed three days after I arrived in America. I went to the hospital frequently. I was having some tonic such as ginseng and deer horn to regain energy after surgery. One day, some of my friends visited to comfort me at home after the surgery and asked me about my health. I responded to them, "I am an old man and it is best to die soon. Don't you think?" Then my daughter-in-law said, "If you want to die so badly, why do you take tonic?" I was shocked and disappointed with her. How could she say that to me? As long as I live, I want to live peacefully and maintain my health in order not to bother others. That is why I was taking some tonic, not because I want to live an extra-long life. In the first place, my daughter-in-law didn't understand me at all and she was not a kind, warmhearted person at all.

We cannot ignore shamanism. I myself remember when my uncle recovered from his leg pains that bothered him every year for a long time. All other treatments and remedies did not work for him except *gut*.* During the *gut* the shaman said that my deceased father caused my uncle's leg pain because my father was not treated with proper care by his family during the preparation for his funeral procession when they hurried to bury him. They didn't even put a Korean stocking on one of his feet. He was properly dressed and buried again very carefully with respect and the proper rituals, and then my uncle healed up completely.

A person at seventy is rusty and, at eighty, useless. It is best to die peacefully without bothering others. I will be eighty-one next year. I have to manage my health while I am healthy. Otherwise, it will be too late. I take Korean traditional medicine made from herbs and animal products once or twice a year. It gives me vital energy and a healthy color to my face. I dye my

---

*A shaman's ceremony to appease spirits and make requests, including healing performed by the shaman through a spirit medium with music, dance, and conversation beyond time and space (Chang, 1996).

hair and put on some lotion. Then I look very young and feel good. Nobody would think I am an eighty-year-old man.

When I reminisce, my recollections are only unpleasant and distressing, which can become very complex and troublesome to me. And then I blow away my worries by smoking—thoughts of the deaths of my two young sons, business failure, maltreatment, loneliness, ill feelings, which make me feel insane. Isn't it a poetic expression? One of my sons died of measles and the other with tuberculosis, which was transmitted by my brother-in-law, who lived with us. I know that smoking is bad for one's health, but the helpful points are greater than the harmful aspects in my situation. If I don't smoke, I think I will go crazy with all the terrible thoughts about my past. Smoking helps me blow away the agonizing thoughts. Otherwise, I can quit smoking any time because I did it before.

It is important to understand the cause of psychological shock and then comfort the person to lift the spirits by providing an opportunity to travel, to drink, to listen to favorite music, to dance, and to spend time with coquettish women regardless of having a wife or not. If people strain their nerves a lot mentally, they develop a lump from hardening of blood and nerve disease.

I feel too lonely to do anything now. I cry alone in the moonlit night. When I am sick, I get lonelier. I feel like I am living in a hell or prison. I am not motivated to live, but I wish to die. As I think of my past, I am smothered by my depressed mood. I have neither a place to go nor someone to talk to. I experience such empty feelings. I try to endure my loneliness by going out and dining out. I go shopping every two or three days. I take a walk on a lonely road as I reminisce and am homesick. But most of the time, I sit around at home. As I endure it, it brings me *shingyungshayak,* nervous disease [neurasthenia]. The nerves [unpleasant emotions] become hard and weakened. I am continuously lonely even now. I went to two psychiatrists and they recommended that I get a girlfriend. However, it is hard to find someone who is compatible with me in terms of education, hobbies, and interests. When I was in Korea, I felt free since I was in my own country, and I did not feel lonely because I had a good time with my friends. I went to movies and traveled. I was healthy. I got along well with my family.

I feel lonely living alone as a widower. I have been a patriarch in an extended family and a man who was not used to taking care of himself alone by cooking, washing, and housekeeping. It is awkward and burdensome for me. Sometimes the dishes I cook taste all right and sometimes they are tasteless.

My friend comes with his car sometimes and we go out together. I went to a Korean Christian church in the past. But these days, I seldom go there. When I go there, we are expected to stay there all day. The chairs are hard and the sermons are long and they do not make sense to me. I used to enjoy writing but these days I cannot concentrate. Anyway, a piece of writing I did was sent to the Korean newspaper, but, strangely, it was not published this time. I'd better check on that.

My life in America makes me depressed. My depressed mood is a symptom, not a disease. I was a very happy, compassionate, and sympathetic man once. The life I am leading is like life in prison. I would like to depart this life as soon as possible if this is the only way I can live. There would be no trouble if I were living in Korea all the time. I have to face troubles with transportation, language, and culture shock. Depression is called loneliness, *hwabyung,* mental illness, or *shingyungshayak*. My disharmonious marital relationship started three days after marriage. My business was a failure in the past and I have to face loneliness every day.

I feel like I am living in a human hell. I feel even more so when I am ill. Unbearable anger and irritability rise up to my head. Tears come down. After crying I feel a little better. Now, even the tears are all dried up. No hope. I barely survive day by day. I worry about how I should spend today and the next day. I feel that every day is a living hell. I frequently feel sad and am in a depressed mood. Frequently the sorrow and depression are very severe. When it is severe, I go out on the lawn and roll around on it. When the depression is moderate, I listen to music and sing. I converse with the canary. When the bird cries, it calms me down emotionally and it makes me feel better. My indigestion and insomnia were severe in the past but I can manage them much better now.

I just want to die quietly if I have to live as I am living, although I really want to live for one thousand years. It is more troublesome to live than to die. Once you are born, you have to die one day. I think of death and I worry about dying. You have to comfort yourself although you curse death.

I become angry, sad, restless, irritable, and my body is weakened. It is called *shingyungjil.* It is a kind of acting-out behavior. It is considered a personality or individual characteristic. These kinds of characteristics are seen among people who have blood type AB. I have blood type AB. The depression is prolonged; I don't think anyone who has a personality like mine will survive. I attempted to kill myself. I thought it was better than to live. One time in the past I collected sleeping pills. Finally I visited a psychiatrist because I thought I was about to go crazy. He told me to get a girlfriend as I already told you. I agreed with him, but it is hard to find a decent woman. I didn't go back to the psychiatrist.

It is how one regulates one's mind. If one does not care for one's own mind, one becomes insane or will die. I fear that I think crazy thoughts and I act crazy. I am worried that my mind will deviate from the normal, and my thoughts and judgment will not be intact. It is painful to restrain myself. It is difficult to bear it and go forward triumphantly in the situation. I tend to question myself. "Do I need to live in this pain all the time?" I become pessimistic. I wish to die.

Depression affects my daily life. I cannot work on anything actively. I give up easily. I am not interested in anything. It makes me give up my life: I make no plans. I do not have the ability to carry out my plans even when I make them. Depression is called an illness of the mind and emotion, neurosis or *hwabyung,* and these are related to indigestion and insomnia.

I suffer from depression because of my fate, although mine is not severe. It is mild now. Only intellectuals are affected by depression. Unintelligent people are not bothered by it. I cannot communicate with the people who are in my apartment building and church because they do not understand me, are not educated well, and are not cultivated.

> I bear and endure it all by myself. It is up to your mind-set. Calm down and soften your mind and then the depression will disappear. Make friends. My friends recommend that I should find a girlfriend or remarry. However, it is difficult to meet a woman who will match me in terms of level of education and emotional maturity, and be compatible. I went to church and am comforted sometimes. I play hide-and-seek by myself among the trees at night. I sing. The birds singing make me feel better. I go out looking around at nature, taking a walk, seeing how people are living, shopping, making friends, or remarrying. I walk along on a small road.

Mr. Moon tended to repeat the same stories, especially the unpleasant experiences. It may be so because he could not forget his agonizing or regretful thoughts and feelings, but they linger and may have even intensified.

Koreans, particularly the elderly, are stereotypically known as stoic and silent, but Mr. Moon was quite expressive emotionally. He studied literature in Japan. He expressed severe loneliness and depression, although lately he says he has a mild depressive mood. He attributed the causes of his loneliness and depression to his unhappy marriage and widowerhood, lack of caring from some of his children, culture shock, and language problems. He tends to be away from his family, but gets public support and is close to selected friends. Some of his children, but not all of them, contact him. Mr. Moon uses nonmedical, individualized self-care methods, except for vitamins, gingko biloba (an aging-control agent), and a traditional Korean tonic to maintain health and sanity. He believes that medication for depression would not work. He creatively mobilizes his holistic and inner resources to make his life bearable and meaningful as much as possible: listening to birds singing, playing hide-and-seek with himself among big trees at night (to avoid being ridiculed and to be free from loneliness), rolling down small green hills, singing, and so on. In the past, some aristocrats and scholars did similar things to amuse themselves and to beat boredom.

Mr. Moon uses public transportation and leads a regular daily life. He is active, functional, and social although he says he is very depressed most of the time. He had a friend who could drive a car, but recently the friend died suddenly. Mr. Moon is doing his best to create a meaningful and balanced life. He does not sound like a major depressive in the biomedical sense. He was not identified as having major depression according to the DIS-III. It could be understood that he is very lonely. He experienced intergenerational conflicts and role reduction in his family. He did not participate actively in the mainstream of American society, although he had various employment experiences and was very active in the civil service in Korea. He is comfortable with his indigenous religion, shamanism. Once he said that proper ancestor veneration would bring healing to people. But other times, he stated that all those spiritual things are created by people for a moral and ethical life.

He is able to evaluate his reality, his strengths as well as his weaknesses, and tries to lead a balanced life. He can feel seriously depressed if he lets himself, yet he can lift his depressed mood with self-care. He says it is mainly how one governs one's disposition. Seeing a psychiatrist is not a common practice among Korean elders, although Mr. Moon consulted one once or twice. It may be related to his educational background, mobility, and ability to pay and obtain information. Mr. Moon uses pluralistic, holistic health systems. He did not go back to the psychiatrist. The physician did not give him medical treatment but social treatment, with which Mr. Moon agrees.

He commented about his smoking habit as a therapeutic and symbolic way of casting off all his anger, rage, regrets, grudges, and hardships. He smokes to "puff away" his unhappiness and loneliness. For example, he described his wife as though she were made of all negative thoughts, characteristics, appearances, and behaviors. She was not flexible enough to change her ways of thinking and behaving to keep up with him. However, he did not divorce his wife because of his children's pleas. Mr. Moon said that he sacrificed himself by not divorcing his wife. Adult Korean children can influence their parents' marriage status sometimes. Although they were not able to have a happy marriage, he said he eulogized his wife on one of the anniversaries of her death because she bore his six children and raised them. As he reminisced, he added that he sympathizes with her very much in his old age. He remarks that she is pitiful and the whole relationship with him is ironic. According to a recent interview, he has been trying to quit smoking with the aid of a nicotine patch.

When his daughter did not let him reiterate what he said about his daughter-in-law, he severely threatened her verbally because she violated the Confucian hierarchy in which the father has the highest authority. She dared to be disrespectful and to not obey her father. Mr. Moon behaved the way he did because his self-esteem was already low even before his daughter responded in a way he did not expect. That is why he was extremely outraged and complained of acute heartaches.

Mr. Moon was pleased with his son's success, especially since the son was influenced by him. Mr. Moon gives himself credit as a wise and kind father in raising his youngest son. He finds happiness among his children, in nature, and through his creative, artful living.

DEPRESSION CAUSED BY HEALTH PROBLEMS

Mr. Won, a teacher, candidly disclosed his multiple health and family problems in relation to his alcoholic sons and his wife, who was subtly expressing unhappiness in their marriage. He related these problems to his lethargy.

> I am a sixty-three-year-old man with a college education and I am a Christian. I taught the Korean language, history, and music. I have five children: two sons and three daughters. I take pleasure in eating food because I do not smoke or drink. In America I worked as a cleaning man.
>
> I feel utterly empty and pessimistic due to my health problems. I have hypertension and diabetes. I had a stroke last year. I usually just smile because I cannot speak clearly, so I have a communication problem. I refrain from going places. The stroke affected my right side, so I cannot even write. My eyesight got worse. My weight was two hundred pounds but now I weigh only one hundred fifty-five pounds. I go to a

medical clinic twice a month and take medication prescribed by my doctor. I can't work and it affects us financially.

I am not hopeful because I feel that I can't accomplish anything. I just maintain the status quo. I really think I am going downhill. I am painfully aware that I can't live long. I regret that I wasn't careful about my health when I was young. I was not careful at all about eating. I hope to and try to live for a long time with my family by controlling my diet and exercising according to my physician's instructions, and trusting in God. I walk for fifteen to twenty minutes a day. I become tired easily, so I have to take a nap. I feel bored, lonely, and empty when my wife goes out.

I achieved everything, such as an education and a profession, all by myself. Nobody helped me. I came to the United States because I wanted to live better by adapting to an advanced country. At the beginning, my wife and I lived with our daughter and now we live in a senior citizen apartment. I realize that whether you are a man or a woman, young or old, you have to work willingly in the United States. In Korea, they respect elderly people, and children provide money and support for their elderly parents. In America, it is not so.

Recently, I am depressed due to the stroke I had. My sons have alcohol problems and they can't adapt to this society. I am very depressed seeing my children who are not useful in the society. Our children don't listen to us. I hope my children become people who are in demand in society and that my wife is strong enough to lead her own life independently. She has backaches due to a "disk."

However, my depression is temporary and momentary. Sometimes I don't even want to speak. If the depression lasts for a long time, death will be inevitable. What I am most concerned about in my depressed state is my death. The death of a parent is natural although it is sad.

Because I am old and sick now, I feel homesick. I want to see my relatives and friends in Korea. I feel isolated from my children. In my youth I had a hobby. Now I can't participate in any activities. It is very hard to receive support or to give assistance to others.

Mr. Won is depressed. He does not seem to be able to integrate his life. He feels that there is a lack of support and pleasurable events within himself and in his environment. His main concerns are his own and his wife's health problems and their sons' alcoholic problems and underachievement. Mr. Won suffers from physical, psychosocial, and spiritual unrest, and he is mostly helpless to solve his own or his family's problems. He worked as a cleaning man although he is a college graduate and former teacher. His depression is related to his health problems, disappointments with his children, his children's uncaring behavior, his wife's disrespectful attitude, his unemployment, the generation gap, and sensing his wife's unhappiness with their marriage.

According to his wife, her husband does not care for her and does not really love her. She says he misses her because he needs her. He is narcissistic, hierarchical, outspoken, and authoritative. He seems to be suffering from his delegitimate state (Kleinman, 1995), as evidenced by a role reduction from his past legitimate, authoritative, and dignified state.

Mr. Won denies having Korean popular illnesses such as *han, hwabyung,* or *shingyungshayak,* but he was sure that he had physical exhaustion. He was able to share his explanation of his health and spiritual problems. He did not use Korean illness idioms to communicate his holistic experience of hopelessness and powerlessness.

PLURALISTIC CARE FOR HOLISTIC HEALTH

Mr. Pyon is a seventy-three-year-old Christian with a primary-school education who has lived in America for six years.

> I worked in a sewing factory and cleaned buildings for one and a half years. I barely live. I have many problems. I have language difficulties, no transportation, health problems, and financial problems. I cannot work because I have "psychogenic hypertension," headaches, and constipation. I always take analgesics and drugs for hypertension. My lungs are bad. I am still alive only because the life span bestowed by heaven is a long one, although I have been near death many times.

My children earned money and we lived together. I didn't educate them, so they don't make enough money. It is my fault. Two years after the independence of Korea from the Japanese occupation, we escaped to South Korea from North Korea. The situation was very bad. I was very much bothered by nerves due to my financial situation. After I failed in business, I sold things on the streets.

I am ashamed of myself. My children went back to Korea. They told me that they wouldn't return to America, so I gave them up by saying, "I cannot stop you if you don't want to return to America where I am."

My parents passed away. My brothers died. My wife died fifteen years ago, and so did my son-in-law with heart disease three years ago. My eldest son had a kidney transplant. My other son gave one of his kidneys to his brother. I grew incompetent in everything. My life is empty. I just blame myself. Who can I blame? I have no more hobbies.

In the beginning when I came to America, I spent time with my friends about once or twice a week. We drank and talked. I am separated from all my friends now. They went back to Korea. I am not feeling good. I feel as though I live in a prison without bars because I cannot work nor do the activities that I like. I have nothing in my hand [no money]. I want to go to Korea but I don't have money.

I am lonely because I don't have a wife. If I was here with my wife and all my children were healthy, I would not have depression. If I could travel with my wife and enjoy things, I would not have depression. I have to be rich. I don't have money. I feel empty. What is the use of living like this? Just being alive is burdensome and irritable. I just think of death. That's why I am depressed. In Korean traditional medicine, depression is also expressed as *hwabyung* or *pung* [stroke] symptoms.

My business failed a long time ago. I had mental shock. I worried a lot about my finances. At that time my parents and brothers passed away. My body became weak and I contracted *shingyungshayak,* from which I have been suffering for forty years. I lost my confidence. If it gets worse, I will go insane and die. When I was about thirty years old, my liver was bad. But I didn't get well, although I was admitted for a year to a renowned medical center in Korea. I also had stewed dried zucchini and mud fish at home and had injections made in Germany. I had analgesics every five hours. I have been continually taking medication for forty years now. It is hard for me to buy my medication because it is very expensive. I had bear gallbladder and it helped me a little with backaches.

I don't show my symptoms of depression to others. I tell them that I have headaches and some leg pains. It is no use telling them about my depression. They might tell me, "You are an old gentleman and shouldn't work. It is too hard on you." The remedies of prevention and healing of depression are a strong will and determination to be positive and joyful. I have to make myself feel good. I took two hundred round little balls of *woohwangchungshimhwan* [an oral medicine made of many kinds of ingredients from herbs, animals, and minerals] but it was not efficacious.

Usually an elderly Korean will say, "I cannot speak, hear, and walk although I have my mouth, ears, and feet!" when they have no transportation and they cannot speak or comprehend English so they cannot go anywhere and cannot meet people to talk to in English. Mr. Pyon uses terms for his condition interchangeably: depression, *shingyungshayak, hwabyung,* heart disease, or stroke, but mostly depression and *shingyungshayak.* He is familiar with depression as a systemic illness of the body and soul. He related his liver ailment to his *shingyungshayak.* He related his illness to the multiple problems of everyday life, widowerhood, relatives' deaths, and separation from his children. He uses various sources for healing and for holistic health.

Mr. Pyon was also affected by sociopolitical disadvantages during World War II and the Korean War. His life and his family members' lives were threatened at that time. He could not educate his children under these circumstances. He is suffering from financial problems and has lost his self-esteem and self-respect. He blames himself for his children's poor financial situation. He takes responsibility, although the sociopolitical situation was very difficult. Education is considered the most important value in Korea. The influence of Confucianism is one of the reasons for this value orientation. He may believe that he has not done enough to deserve his children's filial piety. When his children went back to Korea, he hinted that they did not care for him. He said that he felt a sense of abandonment and rejection and sense of loss of his children even though he appeared to believe the proverb, "One reaps what he sows."

In Korea it is taught that children do not leave elderly and ill parents for any reason. For example, the eldest son is exempted from military duty to care for his elderly parents. Mr. Pyon seemed to conclude that the children's support may not be given when parents do not fulfill their parental duties first. Mr. Pyon expressed sorrow when his children left, although he understood that his children were returning to Korea because they could not make a living in America. He is pessimistic. He misses his deceased wife especially. Not living with his children and his wife makes it very difficult for him to be excited about life when he is surrounded by loneliness. He believes that he is deprived of everything meaningful in his life. He was also diagnosed as having major depression by the DIS-III. His explanation of depression is a biopsychosocial, moral, historical, and traditional medical model. The combination of all his biopsychosocial conditions explains the meaning of his depression, *hwabyung*, and *shingyungshayak*. He did not mention his religious life. His major prescription for his illness is having a meaningful life with significant others and a better financial situation. His catharsis through experiencing Korean illnesses appears to be therapeutic.

Chapter 9

Health, Illness, and Self-Care: "There Is No Caring Son for a Long Illness"

The stories in this chapter relate to health, illness, and patterns of self-care and self-healing mainly based on cosmological, interpersonal, moral, ethical, religious, and spiritual foundations.

A NATURAL PROGRESSION OF LATER LIFE

Mrs. Sin, a sixty-nine-year-old married Christian with a grade-school education, now lives with her husband in a senior citizen apartment. They lived with their children when they arrived in the United States, thirteen years before our interview.

> I have been well since our children obeyed their parents' instructions and studied hard, and they have been well. I have been very busy and happy. I have eight children: three sons (two are elders in church and one is a businessman) and five daughters. I am tired because I have a lot of work to do. I have to take care of my grandsons in my sons' homes and I have to take care of my husband in our apartment. It keeps me very busy to run five houses. I can't help but help my children because they go out to work and their children stay at home all by themselves. It is twice as busy for me in America as in Korea. I get up at five o'clock and awaken my grandchildren, give them breakfast, and send them to school. Then I serve breakfast to my husband and then clean the house. My grand-

children come home from school at two o'clock. I give them a snack and start supper. All of my children live around here in their respective houses. I go around to each of them. I would rather live in Korea than in America, but I stay here to help our children.

On top of that, I study the Bible and English and play the piano. I also play tennis and Ping-Pong. I swim. I am very busy. It is so hard on me now: I am about to die. I don't have any moment to be lonely. In the past, we hired a housekeeper in Korea. Now I do everything by myself.

I had some colds and neuralgia, but they went away after doing exercises. In the past I worried somewhat about my son who had *shingyungshayak*. He studied so hard we didn't know whether he had *shingyungshayak* or not. We thought that he was sick with something else, so we just took him to a hospital. I think he should have been treated differently. I think that he was suffering from some kind of stress. These days I am concerned about my son's business. He spent a huge amount of money on it, but it is not booming.

My vital energy is drained [she is shocked and disappointed or lethargic] after hearing about the nursing home situation in America. My friend visited a nursing home and she was freaked out. When she visited the nursing home she saw that her friends had become skin and bones with malnutrition. They can't digest food or sleep. They are only thinking of going back to Korea. My friend is very depressed because she is worried that she might end up in such a nursing home. She is very anxious to do something to return to Korea because she might end up like her friend in a nursing home if she doesn't. But most of the Korean immigrants don't have anybody or anything in Korea, so, in reality, they can't go back to Korea.

We went to a nursing home. Once we saw the real situation with our own eyes, we couldn't help crying. The nursing home residents were just skin and bones, like ghosts. We cried together with them. They can't even take a proper bath. They are given only a small amount of food to prevent them from having bowel accidents or moving a large amount of feces. They become skin and bones because they can't eat enough when

> they are hungry, although they don't have diseases. After seeing that, all the elderly people become worried and restless and say, "We will become like that in a while. Maybe today or tomorrow because our hearts and eyes are not in good condition." Those who have a son or daughter in Korea want to go back to Korea. Those who don't have anybody in Korea have to stay here. I heard that the situation in a more expensive nursing home is better than in the lower-cost ones. The conditions in the cheapest nursing homes are worst, and the people who work there are worse than animals, and old people are treated worse than animals. All I do is think about how to go back to Korea. When can I go back to Korea? I just think life is empty and I feel sad. I can't forget the miserable nursing home scenes. I become depressed. It won't disappear unless I hear good news. I lost the joy and fun of life. We old people sigh as we say: "We can't help it because that is the reality."

Mrs. Sin worried about her sons when they were young. She still worries about her children's business. There is a Korean saying about having many children: "*Kaji maneun namu param chalnal upda*." (A tree that has many branches will not have moments of stillness undisturbed by the blowing wind.) However, she is able to take it matter-of-factly. One can't be immune to all problems. That is life.

Mrs. Sin seemed to be disturbed by the nursing home situation along with her friends in the original interview. Later, about five years after the original interview, she did not seem to be very concerned about it. Mrs. Sin sounded quite disengaged, although she still makes sure that her grandchildren study. She seems to be less physically involved in housekeeping work. Also, it seems that she has a good chance of living with at least one of her children in America or Korea. Most of the elderly Korean informants are concerned about life at an advanced age with possible disabilities, in particular, those who have poor interpersonal relationships with their children and those who have no savings. According to the informants and their children, elderly and ill immigrants either return to their children or go to nursing homes. Also, when those who are independent become very old, they seem to believe that somehow all things will be taken care of, although they have not made any definite plans for the future. Not many informants talked with their children or others about their plans in case of serious disability or death. It may be so because they leave things to nature. It might be said they are conditioned that way. This kind of attitude may be related to their multireligious cultural backgrounds including Buddhism, Taoism, and shamanism. The informants would usually say, "How can I talk with my children about death?" or something similar, with a tranquil tone of voice. Their children will know what to do for them. Talking about it is not needed and it is understood naturally. Talking only creates awkward interactions, and it is considered indecent.

Mrs. Sin said she doesn't mind whether she is buried in America near her children or in Korea beside her husband. "It will be done by my children. They will do well. I leave it to them," she said calmly. She may have a preference, or she may feel ambivalent about choosing whether to be near her children or her husband. Probably Mrs. Sin decided this way because she doesn't want to burden her children with carrying out her specific wishes. She knows that she likes best what her children will do for her. She added, "My husband was very sure that he wanted to be buried in Korea with his ancestors in our burial ground. It was done according to his wishes." Men seem to be inclined more toward burial near their ancestors and women to their children.

We learned that her husband passed away a year after our second interview, although he had been in good health. She finds herself preparing spiritually for her death, which may come at any time, by reading the Bible, especially Revelation, praying, meditating, and doing things as much as possible to accumulate virtue for the improvement of her karma. She operates her life in the frame of karma, although she is not a Buddhist, because she has lived in the Korean multireligious society.

She helps her grandchildren by advising them to eat properly and study hard. When her grandchildren are big enough to take care of themselves, she believes that they still could be disciplined and cultivated. They can learn Korean directly and indirectly by interacting with their grandmother. She uses the bus and where there are no bus routes, she takes a taxi to her children's houses with her senior citizen discount because her children are too busy to give a ride to their mother. She leads an active life in America. In Korea she might have more leisure and a sedentary life. If given a choice, she prefers the active life and appreciates her sense of achievement and health.

She said when she looks back at her life, she sees that God planned it for her and it went according to God's will, and she is thankful for that. How difficult it seemed for her at the beginning, but God had good ways in the end. She is considered one of the luckiest or most blessed Korean elders. She has children to rely on and she cares for them, and yet she is willing to live and act independently and interdependently with her children.

PHYSICAL ILLNESS CAUSED BY DEPRESSION

Mrs. Shon is a seventy-four-year-old widow. She is a Catholic with no formal education.

> I live with my youngest son, daughter-in-law, and grandchildren. I wanted to move out to a senior citizen apartment but my son didn't allow me to do so. My daughter also lives nearby. I went to her only to work since she owned a sewing factory. I have three other children in Korea. I visited Korea three years ago and I may visit Korea again next year. I live a comfortable life. I eat, have fun, and live with my children. My son and daughter-in-law are devoted and they take good care of me.
>
> In America I can't go around as freely as I did in Korea—no transportation. Suddenly I couldn't see. It was glaucoma that caused my husband's death at age sixty-seven in America. Three years after my husband's death, my eldest son died from hypertension at forty-two. In Korea, my eldest son was known as a good man in our village. He was also talented, learned Chinese characters, and worked in a court. Probably, his fame made his life short. I believe God took my son with him because he was a perfect child. God needed a person like him to do his work.
>
> In America, my eyesight got worse due to my son's death. I can't see very well with glaucoma. I don't want to cook as I

> used to because I'm afraid that some of my hair will accidentally fall in the food. I live with the belief that my eye problem is given by heaven as an inevitable fate. I have sinned and I am in the process of redemption. I had three or four eye surgeries and I am taking medicine. My hands, legs, and feet feel like a sheet of ice and they bother me with numbness. Nothing was wrong with my legs according to the X-rays. I wish I were healthy. Doctors at the hospital I visited told me that I don't have vital energy. It is all depleted because I am old. I worked too hard on our farm to raise my children in my youth, and the doctor added that nothing more could be done except to give me pills for hypertension. My parish church donated money for my son's funeral and our priest visited us almost every day. But I don't remember how I buried him or anything, perhaps because I was in emotional shock. My second son quit his work in Seoul and helped me with our farm work. He is doing well in Korea now.

Mrs. Shon admitted to depression and sadness in relation to her eldest son's death. When children are dead, whether they are young or old, their parents, especially the mother, are traditionally and somewhat symbolically accused of having killed and eaten them up (*jaab a muck da*). It is traditionally believed that they might have abused or neglected their children, that they did not know how to care for them, or that they simply killed them either out of ignorance or intentionally.

"In the beginning, I thought of my eldest son always on a cold day, a rainy day, or while eating." She means that the thought of her son comes to her mind suddenly and frequently whenever something reminds her of him.

> I said to myself, "I have to forget." And then I think of him on his birthday and on holidays. Originally, I was sort of a plain and simple person, and I didn't show tears to others. I cried by myself and struck my chest all by myself. I am always happy in front of others.
>
> In my chest I still can't forget the death of my son. I am in sorrow. Out of nowhere, I think of him and he flits before my eyes, and then I miss him terribly. I pray in front of St. Mary and then I feel better. It is no use to tell it to my other children.

> They would only worry. I am still depressed, some days more than other days. I feel lethargic in my legs and I have a palpitation, which I can even feel myself. It is dark in my eyes and I feel faint and dizzy. I lie down to quiet myself. I go out to expose myself to the wind to cool myself off. I just want to leave this world for the next one. I want to go [die] with my two eyes closed tightly and see my eldest son in heaven. I just want to sleep deeply and that is all. Sometimes I enjoy going outside and looking into the sky endlessly as I chat with a friend.
>
> Sometimes I have an urge to fight someone until I don't want to fight anymore. My son, who lives with me, tells me that if I want to strike someone, to strike his wife, my daughter-in-law. Probably he said it jokingly. Then I asked him, smiling ironically: "Where is such a person who strikes her own daughter-in-law?" I can't do that. In Korea, some of my church friends knew my situation and consoled me with their kind words, which helped me calm down. However, I consider my husband's death, in comparison with my son's death, as part of the fact that we all die one day, and he just passed away sooner than I did.

Mrs. Shon still mourns and grieves for her son, but not for her husband. Generally speaking, it is said that it is much harder for a woman to accept her son's death than that of her husband. Koreans consider children as a mother's own flesh and blood. A husband and wife can become strangers when they are not on good terms. There is a Korean saying for this situation: "When a couple turn their backs to each other, they can become strangers."

Mrs. Shon explained about her illness:

> I have *hwabyung* because my chest was very painful after I lost my eldest son. When I am anxious, "fire" or heat in my body comes up to my head and face with great force, and then I have strong headaches and my eyeballs are very painful, as though they are being pulled out. I have high blood pressure and constipation. Even just now I wanted to read the Bible but I couldn't read even one page. I perspire excessively from my head, so that I know that blood energy goes upward to my

> head. When I go to church, perspiration comes down from my head like rain, so that I feel ashamed and awkward to be around people. I have experienced *shingyungshayak* two or three times a week for fifteen years because my nerves are in such distress, because of my son's death at a young age. I am full of health problems. I have given up on my health. I had tonic medicine prescribed by a traditional Korean physician. I didn't experience any improvement. A person from my village died from *hwabyung,* although the person had taken traditional herbal medicine. I take *woohwangchungshimhwan* [medicinal balls made of ingredients from animals, herbs, and minerals]. When I have a headache, I take aspirin.

Mrs. Shon doesn't distinguish *hwabyung* from depression, *shingyungshayak,* or sadness. She calls depression *hwabyung* and *shingyungshayak*. However, she added that she doesn't know much about depression. More or less the same symptoms were presented for all of the above-mentioned illnesses. She was able to explain her illnesses, such as eye pains, headaches, high blood pressure, and perspiration, holistically in relation to emotional distress caused by separation from her loved ones. Also, she believes that her illness is a way of redemption for her sins. Her spiritual explanation of illness as fate or a way of atonement seems to be related to her Catholicism and multiple Korean religions, including Buddhism and shamanism. The concept of being a sinner comes from Christianity. The hardship of separation from loved ones, the person who has to leave and the one who stays behind, is an element of Buddhism.

Her explanatory model (Kleinman, 1980) of her eye problem is related to the deaths of her husband and especially her son. Their deaths were caused by her sin and she is being punished with eye pain. Meanwhile, her physician's explanation is one of physical hard work in her youth, hypertension, and advanced age. There is a discrepancy between client and healer in understanding illness, as pointed out by Kleinman. How will it affect health care? There might be conflicts in health care practices that require very careful multidisciplinary approaches. Her physician prescribed antihypertensive drugs, and she also took Korean traditional medicine, with which she is familiar and comfortable. As a result she had a pluralistic medical treatment including over-the-counter medicines.

"Nerves" here can be interpreted as a mixture of a sense of loss of a most treasured object, painful and pitiful feelings, anger, sorrow, a grudge, resentment, shame, guilt, and emotional distress in longing for her dead son. According to Korean traditional medical principles, a disharmonious phenomenon is shown in Mrs. Shon's description of headaches, perspiration with fire, cold hands, legs, and feet in *um* and *yang* (negative and positive principles). Mrs. Shon continued:

> I pity myself. I am just old and sick and I have lost all my energy. If I could see, I would work at my daughter's factory and I wouldn't be bored. I should finish [die] in Korea, but I am not sure that it will be realized. My youngest son told me that I can visit Korea, but he wants me to come back to America. My son and my daughter-in-law take care of me. Who else would do that? I receive $300 every month and medical care from the U.S. government, but I feel I don't deserve it, and I feel uncomfortable receiving it. I am very grateful. Even a devoted son can't do better than the regular provision of funds and services.
>
> I feel a lot better these days. I used to feel suffocated and a fire started inside of me. I felt like I had to run outside. These days since I am old, I wait until I calm down by myself. How can I talk about these kinds of things to others? I would be contented if my son would do better with his siding work. It is hard for six of us to live on his meager income. I regret that we came to America. My daughter-in-law doesn't say anything, although I shout at my children to release the fire inside of me.

Yet Mrs. Shon seems to be content because her daughter-in-law does not talk back or behave in other unfilial ways. Mrs. Shon feels that she is fortunate. She is thankful for her family's health, although they are not well-off. She feels good about her independence, freedom, and mobility, which are related a great deal to her general health, and the understanding, support, and cooperation of her children. As for her health, she wants to be reassured by medical professionals, although she has her own opinion on matters of health and illness.

In Korea, when a person achieves distinction, people believe that evil spirits will harm him or her out of jealousy. Thus, some people, especially an only son when he is young, are given so-called unworthy names to prevent harm by supernatural evil forces. For example, someone might be called a pig or a similarly unrefined or unvalued name. It may be to teach people modesty and humility. Mrs. Shon interprets her son's death in relation to folk beliefs, and she may believe that if he had been given such a name, he might not have died. In terms of her Catholic faith, she believes that it was an act of God. She eulogized her son. This way she can glorify her son, have peace of mind, and maintain her health.

By using Korean illness idioms, Mrs. Shon was able to talk about her tragic life. At the same time, she was proud of her son and was making her body and mind healthy and peaceful through Korean folk syncreticism and Catholic and Buddhist atonement.

HEALTH THROUGH INDEPENDENCE

Mr. Seo saw elderly Korean people as having *hwabyung*, but he denied having *hwabyung* himself, although he was diagnosed with major depression. Mr. Seo is a sixty-two-year-old widower with a middle-school education, who worked as a fireman for the U.S. Army in Korea for thirty years. He was healthy in Korea. He came to America one year before his retirement and worked in a laundry owned by his daughter. Recently he had a stroke. However, he can do activities of daily living on his own.

According to Mr. Seo, elderly Korean immigrants suffer from *hwabyung* because they expect their children to support them as in earlier times, based on traditional values of filial piety, which require adult children to support and please their parents as they need and wish. However, their expectations cannot be realized and they develop *hwabyung* from the disappointment. Mr. Seo said:

> Adult Korean children in America cannot support their parents like in the old days, although they want to observe filial piety, because they have to leave their family at home and go to

> work. However, most of the elderly Korean immigrants do not understand what hardships their children are going through. They just feel sorry for themselves and have feelings of betrayal, rejection, disappointment, and loneliness. Some of the elderly people feel ignored, frustrated, angry, and depressed, like children. Some blame their children for lack of support and attention to them, although their children try to do their best. Some of the parents suffer from *hwabyung*. Distress of the emotions and mind usually interferes with bodily functions and conditions. Naturally, various diseases will develop, such as indigestion, due to stress. One's life span will be shortened. *Hwabyung* is also called inner illness.

Mr. Seo stated that parents should do everything possible to be independent from their children. He continued that Korean elders should realize that there are environmental, socioeconomic, and value changes and, in spite of these changes, they should learn to become adaptive, content, and happy.

> Loneliness is worse than *hwabyung* and should be overcome by finding pleasant activities and work and carrying them out. Nobody can do it for them. They themselves have to do it. Otherwise, one cannot live long. They have to learn to drive, although their children say they cannot do that because their parents are too old to drive. Indeed, elderly people should insist on driving. If their children are dutiful, they have to buy their parents a big used car. What is more comfortable than that? The elders will become healthy and well immediately because they can go anywhere they like. All illnesses will go away and they will be very happy indeed. In order to become filial children, they have to provide "feet" [a car] for their parents.
>
> I go to the Evergreen University for old people and spend each day without feeling lonely. My wife died ten years ago from hypertension, and it was sometimes difficult to raise our children by myself. It wasn't really too bad because my children did really well and I was paid a good salary. It has been hard since I had a stroke last May. I try not to be depressed by thinking happy thoughts.

The people who come to a senior university seem to be doing all right. But others are lonely. They don't have any problems to get three meals a day, but they are having a hard time because they are lonely. Some of the elders returned to Korea because they would rather spend time with their friends there. They said: "There is no joy in America. How can I live here in America? It is like living in a prison. Wherever I go I have to depend on others." They cannot go out. It is the social structure or way of living here. They live in a senior citizen apartment and if they cannot move around there, then they go to a nursing home. If they cannot adapt there, they blame their sons and daughters. But their children are busy working, so they cannot give more support to their parents, although they would like to do more for them. It is no place to live if you think about it. The social environment is made that way. They cannot speak or go anywhere on their own. They have no friends. It is true.

Their desperate condition can be interpreted in this way: the body is seen as a reflection of the mind, as one system. Powerlessness or helplessness is not only what one feels but also what one actually experiences with one's body. Koreans are from one race so that wherever they go in Korea, everybody can be considered your friend or relative, but not here in America. Some stubborn elders, who strongly feel that they did their best for their children, are still expecting their children to do everything they need, but it cannot be done because their children have to go to work to survive.

I know an old gentleman who is seventy-eight now. He learned to drive when he was seventy-seven although his children discouraged him. He goes everywhere with his wife and they say, "There is no place like America." Although they do nothing, they receive welfare money the first day of each month. What son or daughter would do that? They said they are so happy to live in paradise on earth although they are old.

Most of the other elderly people do not have the courage to be independent and so they feel lonely. Their feelings are disturbed, stress accumulates, and then diseases and illnesses develop. They cannot move around; then they get headaches and backaches. They age quickly and their life span shortens. They just wait for the day when they will die. Elderly Koreans are lonely because they feel depressed and angry because, naturally, they tend to think their children neglect them. It gets worse because they have immigrated to a new environment. Their depression could be *hwabyung*. Some elderly parents are not satisfied with the amount of filial behavior that their children render and they feel betrayed and rejected. They express their hurt feelings in various ways. Some of them even go berserk in the worst situations.

They only have thoughts of death. They say it is much better to die than live like that in old age. They are just living because they are alive. There is no meaning in living like this. Although they are elderly, they should lead a meaningful and joyful life. But it is not so, sot they don't want to live. They are depressed and they sigh and they wish they could go back to their homeland. But in Korea, there is nobody waiting for most of them, and there is no place for them to live because they sold their properties and most of their family and relatives came to America.

The elderly Korean adults who live in the apartments that were built by the Korean Association are having fun. They can communicate with other Koreans there. Depression cannot be cured by medication. Tranquilizers make people's minds cloudy. They need some programs to relieve their stress. Parties may help them too. Going to church once a week helps them to lift their spirits by meeting their family and friends and listening to a sermon. People have to decide by themselves to be happy and overcome depression. They have to make plans to do meaningful, fun things. Others cannot do much for them. They have to be motivated to be active and independent. Then they will get better and healthier right away. All the illnesses or diseases will disappear. In order to be devoted to their parents, children should help their parents by driving them places, as they like. It is the priority.

Mr. Seo explains loneliness, depression, or *hwabyung* in relation to aging, immigration, and psychosocial dynamics between parents and children. This is an objective, valuable, peer observation of the reality of elderly Korean immigrants and their children. It strongly recommends taking opportunities for enhancing mutual understanding between them. There should be no room for self-pity, complaining, blaming, resenting, or being regretful among elderly Koreans. Mr. Seo thinks that adult Korean children should teach and help their parents with self-care as much as possible so that their parents will become self-sufficient and independent and maintain harmonious relationships with their children.

LIVING COURAGEOUSLY AND PATIENTLY

Mrs. An, sixty-eight, is married and has a high school education. She came to America in 1976. She has one son, two daughters, and one son-in-law. She is a patient and self-sufficient grandmother.

> Recently, I began staying at home and doing housework, cooking, caring for my grandchildren, and gardening except when I go to church. My eyesight is bad. It is a big problem when I study the Bible. Most of the time I was comfortable in Korea, although I was sick sometimes. I spent time with my friends and visited many places with them. Living in America for old people is like hell. But, if you take your troubles to Jesus, all your problems are solved. I experienced many more psychological and emotional troubles in America than in Korea, although material conditions are better in America than in Korea. Language problems made me angry and distressed quite often. However, when a mediocre foreigner picked on my English with arrogance, I defended myself pretty well because I have a strong mind. Because of my poor English, my coworkers looked down on me and I threatened them with tae kwon do kicks and they did not bother me any longer. I wanted to go back to Korea but I overcame it with patience. I am not depressed because I comfort myself with the Bible. Of course, depression is just a state of mind.
>
> When a person is not self-confident and not faithful to God, depression comes on. A person with depression does not have her normal mind, but that of a psychotic person. Her behavior

is odd. Her thinking is not clear and she thinks of something idiosyncratic. She gets depressed even if she feels a little bad. She feels like it is a rainy day. She cannot face the world boldly because she becomes anxious in mind and in body. If she cannot have peace of mind, she gets depressed. Depression is related to family and daily life. Most of the people go on with their lives, even though they are depressed. But it is troublesome, if they do not have mental power. Depressed people have weak minds.

I am usually full of fun and energy. When I am about to be depressed, I tell myself I should not be that way and I bounce back. Although I do not like to do certain things, I push myself to do them, and then I could do well. In the past, when I was depressed, I tried to have good thoughts and I got together with my friends. Now I read the Bible and meditate. The way to prevent sadness and depression is to know oneself in relation to the troubled situation, whether it is originated by oneself or by others, and overcome it by solving it. If you cannot solve it, you have to help yourself accept it with understanding and peace of mind and harmony for yourself and others.

If people don't intend to show others sadness and depression and conceal them, others have no way of knowing it. They can keep them inside of themselves. There is no way that others can find out about it. If they let others know their sadness and depression, then even others will be affected by it. They should not make others sad and depressed with their dysphoric mood. If they do, it is committing a sin as a Christian and they should feel guilty about it.

By the way, sadness and depression are nerve symptoms related to *hwabyung*. Any illness can bring complications if one is not careful with one's health. According to my careful observation, *hwabyung* or *woolhwabyung* sufferers are hot-tempered, irritable, and narrow-minded. *Hwabyung* occurs when people try to achieve what they want by relying only on their own stubbornness instead of inviting nature's way and other people's ways. These kinds of people cannot lead a satisfactory life. They may have to face grave situations if they do not understand their problems and do nothing about them.

> They have to be honest with themselves and others in daily life and heal themselves. They have to eliminate their stupid thinking of "I am sad. I am depressed" and act wisely. Like any situation, after all, the cure originates in one's mind. One has to cultivate one's mind.

Mrs. An reminisced about her unpleasant immigration experiences—in particular, her language problems at work—which were difficult enough to cause her to suffer from depression. But, with a sense of humor, she described how she triumphed over instead of being swallowed up by depression or *hwabyung*, by using self-defensive and offensive tactics, and holistic strategies. They are a combination of tae kwon do (a Korean martial art) and a cultivated mind. She has a detailed explanation of depression in relation to human nature, origins, phenomena, prevention, and self-care as she connects depression with Korean folk illnesses through her experience and the life experiences of others. She understands depression as a bizarre emotional, psychotic phenomenon of cognitive disturbance that affects a person and his or her family's whole life. Still, she believes that one can control depression. Thus, the sufferer can be perceived as an average, normal person. Mrs. An does not seem to believe in the objective nature of the phenomena of depression.

She believes that ethically and morally people should keep a depressed mood and behavior to themselves to protect themselves from the stigma and to protect others from becoming depressed.

She seems to be concentrating more on spiritual life as she gets older. She recognizes inevitable physical deterioration such as poor eyesight, which hinders her reading of the Bible. Mrs. An sends the message that a cultivated, mature, and sound mind disciplined in nature and religion is essential for harmonious relationships with oneself and others.

THE TASKS OF OLD AGE

Mrs. Chin is a sixty-seven-year-old married theological-school graduate who has lived in the United States for twenty-three years. In contrast to most of the other elderly Korean immigrants, who live either by themselves in senior apartments or with their adult children, Mrs. Chin lives in her own house with her family. In addition, Mrs. Chin and her husband came to America by themselves through his employment as an engineer, while most of the immigrants were invited by their adult children.

> My husband easily obtained his job in America. For the first three years, I felt strange and lonely in America. Soon we felt all right because we have lived a Christian life. We forgot our loneliness by working hard at our church and at work. I was tired because I worked very hard. In America, we are very busy. I don't understand why we have to be so busy. I feel like I am in an industry where human beings are eugenically engineered for doing work. I feel like we don't earn much money commensurate with the hard work we do. I feel like I just work hard without enough reward. In Korea, all I had to do was oversee family affairs, but here in America, I actually work to earn money for the first time in my life. Besides, in Korea we had lots of people who helped us. All in all, the hard work we do in America is nothing compared with the hardships experienced during the Korean War. Our house was destroyed. Our bodies, minds, and souls were fatigued while we were escaping to South Korea. When we arrived in South Korea, my husband and I had to build our own house.
>
> I am an open-minded person, so I don't get depressed easily. I am determined to overcome difficulties and I trust God, who helps us. I believe in God and I am just waiting to die because I have lived long enough. I don't think I can get *hwabyung*, depression, or *shingyungshayak.*
>
> I want to rest a little. I want to sell our laundry business and rest. Also, my eyes are not good. I had eye surgery. I am going to spend more time in church. I have some difficulty with language but, actually, it is not a big problem for me as long as I don't get frightened. My family helps me with transportation.

Mrs. Chin recognized the differences between an easy, leisurely life and a busy, hard life, and appreciated the memories and reminisced about them. She believes that she has a resilient character and personality to endure any hardships because of her faith in God. She wants to take care of her health and have time for spiritual devotion in the final stage of her life, which she set as a priority in her mind early in her youth. She seems to have the resources, flexibility, and wisdom to know when to stop one phase of life and freely choose another more appropriate venture that interests her.

EMOTIONS EXPRESSED AS PHYSICAL ILLNESS

Mrs. Yong, a sixty-one-year-old high school-educated housewife, has struggled to control strong emotions related to *hwabyung, han,* alcoholic sons, and an unsupportive husband. She says she is on the way to spiritual healing.

> I have *hwabyung* due to my inner injury [upset, emotional distress, conflicts, anger, and frustration]. My inner injury has been very severe to cause *hwabyung.* I have been depressed continuously, every day, for a long time. When others tell me something unpleasant or they ignore me, although it would be ordinary to others, sometimes it feels like a thorn. When someone tells me something unpleasant, I feel it like a dagger stuck forcibly into my chest.
>
> I cannot accept favorably what others say. I tend to hear it negatively instead of positively. It is a big problem for me that I cannot digest what others say. I get dizzy in my head and vomit easily. I know it is a health problem. I have a personality of fire, so I become easily enraged although I am a woman (I was taught that a woman shouldn't be like that but should be restrained and submissive). If I am able to behave the way I want to, I will be fine, but I cannot do that most of the time. Then I get frustrated and depressed. I would like to strike the cheeks of the people who make me angry, but I cannot do that. I have to be patient because I am a woman. I cannot digest the anger, which is why I am in pain. I lose myself and I give up. I don't gain anything that way. Also, I get depressed when my children do not listen to their parents' advice, but behave the opposite way. What I say is not understood by others or is ignored.
>
> Then, shockingly, I get enraged and tearful and want to cry forever. My whole body gets numb and I cannot move freely. I

do not have enough strength to hold even a piece of paper. I do not feel good and I become very tired mentally and physically. Then I lie down and cannot eat anything. Ultimately it harms my body and ruins my health. I lose myself and I give up on myself. Nobody can help me except God.

I have diabetes mellitus, arthritis, and heart disease with symptoms of heart attack, hypertension, and facial paralysis. I feel my head is too heavy to hold. I cannot control when I am enraged, so I behave roughly. And then I regret it immediately. I try to overcome it with faith and prayer but sometimes the rage just comes out. When others talk about me, it makes me feel that a knife comes and intrudes into my chest so that I tend to reject it. It may even endanger my life. I cannot digest what others say to me; it is a big problem. Again, it is a big problem that I cannot be patient. I try to console myself. Talking to a person like in this interview really helps me. I feel really happy right now.

Mrs. Yong vividly explained her psychogenic pain in physical terms. She is trapped in her distress and she cannot seem to regulate and release it. She feels that she has no one to talk to and no one who can understand her in her environment.

I have had *han* all my life since my marriage. My selfish husband and two sons, who live by drowning in alcohol and depending on their parents financially, are the main reasons why I have *han.* I was most sad and depressed when my husband did not understand me and my youngest son was drowning in liquor. After he drinks alcohol, he physically strikes his family and asks for money.

In ordinary times I feel calm, but when situations arise, I get anxious and nervous. If a person whom I don't like is not there, my frustrations disappear, but if a person I don't like is there, I immediately flare up fiercely. Then I explode in a rage. I cry out for God. I feel relieved after I have a flood of tears. I think my faith is growing.

I dreamed of a beautiful marriage and expected to raise my children perfectly. I am very disappointed with our marriage and our children's behavior.

> *Han* destroyed my health. The *han* was severe enough that I felt like I was dying. It is painful to have *han*. My life closed in on me while I was suffering from *han*. If *han* is prolonged, I will not be able to recover from diseases. The only treatment to heal my *han* is singing hymns and praying. Then I will appreciate the meaning of life and I will be glad. *Han* is also called a knotted mind.
>
> When the *han* started, there was high anxiety and a warlike tension in my family. The *han* caused me to lose my motivation, hope, and aspirations for life and give up my plans. The *han* affected the health of my body terribly. It made it difficult to bear life problems. Sometimes I could not fulfill the role of caring, dutiful, and responsible mother.

Mrs. Yong described her unique meaning of *han* as shame and guilt: "I didn't do any harm to others outside of the family. They do not know that I have *han*. So far I sacrificed myself, with everything I have, for my children and husband. My husband was a gourmet. I tried to cook everything he likes by doing research."

She believed that she sacrificed and devoted herself to others. She thought that as long as she did that, everything would be all right with her and she would be contented and satisfied. Later she found out that that was not true. She added, "From now on, I will go my way with God's will." Park (1995) stated that any meaningful religion helps people to save their spiritual and meaningful existence, which cannot be accomplished in any other way. Mrs. Yong called her condition *hwabyung* but later she started to call it *han*. She used the terms interchangeably.

In her case, *han* could mean agony and distress caused by an unfulfilled dream. She set out with high expectations for her marriage and children. However, she does not think that these were realized. Although she tried very hard, her philosophy and practice of collectivism seem to be transformed into those of individualism after her dream did not come true. Still, she puts a high priority on her family.

Mrs. Yong spoke Japanese. She worked in a Japanese restaurant. She stated:

> I wasn't lonely, but glad when I was working. However, it brought me nothing but diseases and illnesses. I couldn't work due to my health problems and, really, I have been feeling that I am useless, empty, and lonely for five or six years now. When it is severe, my tears roll out endlessly. When sadness overwhelms me, I cry tearfully. The sadness induced by my children is greater than that from the death of my beloved mother because I became ill from my children's troubles. I depend on my religion. I regain my strength and motivation by praying, singing hymns, and talking with God. What I gained from my experiences of anger and depression is faith in God and living by the rewards of Jesus Christ.

She stated that the crucifixion of Jesus Christ gives her courage to overcome problems and live happily. She feels embarrassed to complain about her hardships in comparison with Jesus' pain. She started the interview by saying, "My life in old age is vain and empty." Mrs. Yong said that she felt that her husband and children exploited her. If she strikes back or gets even with her husband and children, she will be stigmatized because of the idea that a woman and mother should not behave that way. She feels that this is a no-win situation for her. She cried, "I have only an aged and diseased body. I thought I would live forever. But it is in vain." She expressed her profound despair. She admitted that her personality causes her trouble and she does not have a confidant. When her husband was interviewed, he did not mention her distress, although he knows about her health problems. Korean women learn that they should show only happy faces and say pleasant things (Kim, 1975) whether or not they are happy inside. However, Mrs. Yong admits that she cannot control her anger. She tries to control her emotions with faith. She said, "I hope that if my children could not be filial children, at least they wouldn't cause anger and frustration in me. When I treasure my God in my soul, then I live. I just follow my God."

She and her Korean traditional physician made a diagnosis of *hwabyung*. She believes that the illness threatens her life. Her symptoms were described as sensitive and irritable nerves (worries, frustrations, anger, and irritability) and a psychogenic nature—*shing-*

yungjil jurk igo shingyungsung i da (irritable nature and nerve symptoms, according to her Korean traditional physician). She also has been treated with herbal medicine and acupuncture. Crying seems to relieve her frustrations. Her faith in God heals her.

At the end of the interview, she said:

> Because I am a woman, if I say something even a little more than necessary, I am sure I will be immediately told that I am too talkative, although I talk truthfully. Now, I feel really well, as though I have breathed a rush of fresh air after a long, unbearable suffocation. I feel the anger inside has been relieved after I have talked about everything inside of me.

She was utterly disappointed with the reality of her "indifferent husband and sons drowned in alcohol." That may be why it was so hard for her to find equanimity, along with her emotional, easily hurt nature and her unrealistic expectations.

In her late stage of life, she seems more individualistic than collectivistic, which might be related to the fact that she has been living in America. Her holistic ideals of exchange with family members did not happen according to her wishes and perceptions. She is exhausted. She said that she has to go her own way for her physical health and her sanity.

Her language demonstrates the somatization of social and emotional problems, for example, "I cannot digest what others say." When she hears, feels, or sees something unpleasant, it is transformed into anger, then depression. It stays in her body and is expressed as a disease.

In the most recent interview with her, she said she has been able to enjoy peace of mind and lead a grateful life thanks to God. She recognized that she and God have a mutual and cooperative relationship and she is also much more tolerant with her sons. In the Korean idiom, she has been cultivating herself by slowly gaining insight and truth about her life. She added that her health has improved. Through spiritual awareness and practice, she has been transforming herself into a more emotionally tolerant and healthier, well-rounded individual, although she admits that she is still labile at times. She may represent women in transition from male-dominated hierarchical collectivism to individualism. She feels that her sense of self as an individual was not respected. She was seen as a permanent nurturer for others, but never for herself. She sees herself as victimized, for example, by a male-dominated family and society. Finally, she found the comfort that she has been seeking from her family from Christian religion. It helped her to be more tolerant and understanding of her family and herself.

RECOVERY FROM ABUSE THROUGH SELF-CULTIVATION

Mrs. You, who is sixty years old and has an elementary-school education, stated that *hwa (hwabyung)* leads to *shingyungshayak*. Mrs. You used the names of Korean folk illnesses interchangeably. She has many grudges against her husband because of his extramarital affairs and his self-centered lifestyle.

> My husband always does the opposite from me. We are not compatible at all. It gets worse as the days go by. I did not know that he could be that bad. How could he go around and have a pleasurable time with married women when I was twenty-six to thirty years old? I have lived to get revenge on him for his unbelievably horrible, ugly, and cruel treatment of my children and me. He was possessed by evil so that he abused and tortured me. My husband is a hypocritical, self-centered, and weird man, who had mental problems, and was admitted to a psychiatric hospital in America. He was kind to everyone except me. Whenever he saw me, he beat me up. My body was all bruised. I lost my soul [fainted] when my husband was pulling me around after beating me [nearly] to death. I thought I was dying. I tried to kill myself by taking medication but failed.
>
> He took all the money from me and ran away from home at a very important and financially hard time for our children. He did not provide anything financially. I had such a hard time feeding our children. I worried that our children might die of starvation. However, I didn't even think of asking for assistance lest our dignity should be torn from us. I came up with the idea of killing us together, my son, my daughter, and

> myself. My son disagreed with that but my daughter agreed. I had to give up the idea of killing us.
>
> I had to fight on the front line of survival. I worked as a peddler, an insurance broker, and a saleswoman at a beer store. Finally, my husband lost all his money and returned home. A while later he gathered everything that had monetary value and left again. At that time I attempted the "accompanied suicide" with my children. Suicide is a terrible thing to do as a mother. Children should not die before their parents do. But, there was no other way I could think of. Again, I was thinking about suicide, but I did not attempt it because it is a sin to commit suicide before my parents passed away. One time he told me that if I lived with my children, he would not provide living expenses, so I lived separately from my children for two years. Now he is being punished. Our children do not respect him. I even had homicidal thoughts about him.
>
> I had frequent abortions. It was very painful when "husband-wife physical relations" took place. He had extramarital affairs. We were divorced. After he finished his affairs with two other women, he asked me to get back together again. I agreed to it for our children's sake. From the beginning of our marriage, he had hepatitis, and he transmitted it to me. I have *han* [grudges, sadness, regret, and resentment] in my mind. In the first place I did not want to get married but wanted to go on to higher education, but my parents forced me to get married. I wanted to come to America alone without him accompanying me, but our daughters-in-law in Korea avoided him and did not care for him, so we had to bring him with us. I live with my daughter so I can look after my grandchildren and help her with the housekeeping. My husband lives in a subsidized senior citizen house by himself.

Mrs. You expressed her concerns about her children. Her daughter failed in her business and also does not have a good marital relationship. Her son-in-law is narrow-minded and not motivated, according to Mrs. You. Her daughter has to motivate her husband. Mrs. You's son was "doing labor," which is not considered a respectable and secure occupation. She said, "That is why my mind is painful. He does labor because he could not speak English. He is thinking about going back to Korea." She also experienced numerous family deaths. Mrs. You continued:

> I had very severe insomnia every night when I had *hwabyung* and *shingyungshayak* because you cannot forget resentments or worries. I had feelings like suffocating inside and fire flaring up in my chest. It developed this way: first I had indigestion and then the fire started inside when I stayed at home, then I had to run out. I always had headaches and coughs. I had stomach trouble, heart disease, painful urination, and three operations for sinusitis. My head became soft and it was throbbing. The back of my head was pulling. I had darkness in my eyes. My hands and feet were becoming numb and had a bluish color. Injuries of the mind and soul with internal or mostly external origins seem to cause physical diseases in major organs. I had a strong heart [usually the mind and soul] but it became weakened while I was defending myself from my husband's torture. It is the same principle. If a storm hits a tree hard, the tree will break and fall.
>
> My life was so tragic. I tried to kill myself in the sea. But it was difficult. One of my friends killed herself with one of her children in the sea. I had not only suicidal thoughts, me alone without my children, numerous times, but also I had homicidal thoughts of killing my husband with a hammer, who, when he came home after drinking, broke everything in the household, and then took a nap. When depression gets worse, one could kill oneself or harm others.
>
> Probably I committed many sins in my previous life and my fate is ugly. I wanted to cry and I did that too much. There are different manifestations of these phenomena. I felt that I was insane. When nobody was around, I wanted to sit absentmindedly, endlessly. However, because I have a well-rounded personality without too many angles [an understanding, flexible, open, and generous mind], I could persevere, tolerate, and overcome the unbelievable conditions. I know there were many men who had extramarital relations and had concubines. One of my friends had *hwabyung*. She had a fever and was

paralyzed all over her body. At last she died of *hwabyung*. I realized that *hwabyung* was dreadful.

Depression, *hwabyung, shingyungshayak,* and *gasm ari* [chest illness] are related and are the same. I experience *hwabyung* whenever I see my husband. Fire comes to the body and it becomes *shingyungshayak.* The body becomes bad because of fire. The kidneys are affected and then it goes to the lungs. Fire is not good for the kidneys. One could become an idiot or insane person. I experienced it. I have had *hwabyung* since my husband played around with other married women. I could not sleep due to *hwabyung* or *shingyungshayak*. He disappeared with the money that he got for selling the ship we had in order to gamble with his women. At that time I had nothing and became a beggar.

I rely on my religion. Previously I blamed my parents, my husband, and others for my bad fate. When I did not have religion, I gave up everything. However, *nammihoranggaenggyo* [a Buddhist-related religion] teaches that all troubles and pains come from the self. When I was reborn from death, I was covered with rust, and if I brush it off and polish away the dust with devotion, faith, and self-cultivation by accumulation of virtue, I will be at peace.

I have been devoting myself ardently to *nammihoranggaenggyo.* I read its scriptures and chant *kyung* [a selected portion of Buddhist scriptures] in front of Buddha. It helped me. If I did not have religion, I would have been dead a long time ago. I yield myself to understanding the principles of Buddhism. I try not to hate my husband although he abused me physically, psychologically, and spiritually, and battered me because it was my fate. A person makes his or her own happiness or misfortune. It all depends on how you make up your mind. I have become patient and I do not talk back when people insult me for no reason. I always live as if I don't count in dealing with others.

Koreans are taught to yield to others as much as possible. They give others a chance and they give in to others. They do not defend themselves lightly in embarrassing situations in order not to lose face. They put themselves in a lower position than the other person.

Mrs. You also carries an amulet made of rice paper with a red colored stamp. Such amulets, usually in Chinese characters, ask supernatural powers to protect the wearer, his or her family, and others from evil or disease. Religious and cognitive awareness and support from her children gave her solace. She continued:

> These days my children are very good to me. I don't let others know about my problems. The few people who know about my problems said that I was in a sad situation or I was courageous. But I did not tell them everything including the homicidal thoughts although I was in a life-threatening situation many times. I feel good these days. For the first time in my life, I have told you about my concealed emotions and sad personal history, which were difficult for me to hide.

Sometimes *hwabyung* is explained as an acute disease with involvement of all systems of the body, manifested by paralysis, idiocy, insanity, and fever. *Hwabyung* is directly related to the cognitive and emotional domain, according to Mrs. You's explanation: "I experience *hwabyung* whenever I see my husband." To Mrs. You, her husband was the representation of the worst evil in the whole cosmos. *Hwabyung* was explained as a conditioned response to her horrible lifelong experience with her husband. Mrs. You was able to explain her *hwabyung* experience with Korean medical ideas about fire, the lungs, and the kidneys in a systematic, synthetic, and holistic way.

She claims that she was able to survive because of her tolerant personality, tenacity, religion, and ability to control her mind and thinking. Suffering from *hwabyung, han,* and/or *shingyungshayak* is an experience that symbolizes the most tragic and difficult human conditions. At the same time, they can be healing and one can become a saint like Mrs. You through an enduring cognitive and emotional process, self-cultivation.

Mrs. You accepts as karma all the hardships and distress in her life. She thought that it was her husband who tortured her, but she realized that her fate or her previous life was responsible. However, this is no dead end for her, but an opportunity for peace of mind.

She has conquered her fate and won peace with herself, her husband, her family, and others through cultivating herself and accumulating virtues through her religion.

KEEPING FAITH AND HIGH MORAL STANDARDS OF CONDUCT TO DEFEAT DEPRESSION

Mrs. Back, sixty-five, is married and has a college education. She originally came to America to study and has lived in the United States for forty years. She prays and consults a physician to recover from her stroke, which occurred several years ago. Following her stroke, she has been depressed, as she is disabled.

> I really prayed hard to overcome the stroke. I thought it was unfair to have to suffer from it, because we had bought a house after our long, hard work and effort, and we were about to enjoy living in the house. Suddenly, I had to suffer from a stroke. At that time, nothing pleased me, and it was like losing myself. However, my most sincere and earnest prayer helped me to revive myself from the distress. I was in a depressed mood, but I was not depressed psychopathologically.
>
> People who have depressive illness are immature fools and weaklings. They have a narrow personality and cannot regulate their frustrations. If they were sound and well-rounded, they would never develop depression. They have depressive illness because they do not have faith. Depression grows where trust and dependability are lacking. If depression is prolonged, people lose humanness, self-esteem, and health. They die gradually as they do not know God's power. Sometimes a whole family will be broken and saddened if people cannot be good mothers and fathers.

Mrs. Back explained depression from a holistic, moral, and psychosocial point of view. Also, it is not a matter of the individual but the whole family who have the potential to affect a whole village with depression. She continued:

> When I am sad, I pray and meditate. I was filled with anger, distress, and depression, but they were removed by my pray-

> ing. I asked God for forgiveness and I was saved. If one talks with God directly, all problems will be solved, and one will gain strength. Diseases, illnesses, or sicknesses will be treated by God's love. If people have generous minds, they will overcome depression with patience. In order to get rid of depression, people have to understand themselves and boldly wake themselves up from a leisurely, easy life. I do not care what others think of me as long as I know that I am doing all right.

Mrs. Back's sense of self is strong. According to her, depression is caused by one's lack of faith, dysfunctional state of health, and a narrow-minded personality. She described depression almost as addictive and an intoxicating indulgence. In other words, depressed behaviors are uncultivated character traits and behaviors. Also, personal feelings and perceptions of lack of support from family members at the time of illness or vulnerability seem to contribute to the construction and explanation of depression, along with the individual's personality and the difficulty of the situation.

Mrs. Back's self-care methods are having faith, praying, and asking for forgiveness for her sins. She does not discuss physical complaints, although she appears to be uncomfortable and restrained. She is obviously making serious efforts to maintain socially expected emotional and moral decorum by self-cultivation and religious faith. When she was contacted again a few years after the first interview, the conditions caused by her stroke had become worse. She was very uncomfortable and irritable with her condition, to the degree that she refused to be interviewed again.

Chapter 10

At Last, Death: Can a Person Really Want to Die?

In this chapter, stories about the last life event are presented. Some of the very old Korean elders said that they were ready to pass away naturally and peacefully.

DISENGAGEMENT OF KOREAN ELDERS

Mrs. Song is an eighty-five-year-old married Christian who lives with her second son. She has had eye surgery. Another son died about ten years ago, and her daughter died about fifteen years ago. Mrs. Song said, "I was pitiful and in great pain. I tried to forget the tragedy by myself because it wasn't something to tell others. But I didn't give up anything in my life." When Mrs. Song thinks of her children, particularly her son, she is sad and lonely. Having a son is absolutely necessary in Korean society. Sons are traditionally responsible for supporting their parents and venerating ancestors. She said her loneliness is not so severe now. Sometimes she has indigestion.

Her buffer against depression might be that she is relatively healthy, at her advanced age, being married, living with her children, and having religion. She has an easygoing, understanding, and accepting personality with a caring manner, so she does not worry. She knows that she cannot do much for her children in her old age although she is concerned, especially when they have problems.

Through a recent contact, I learned that she is suffering from neuralgia in her thighs and legs. She used to take many kinds of medication, but they were not effective. These days she is not taking any medications. Her husband is a ninety-six-year-old Presbyterian minister, who gets up at five o'clock in the morning to pray and read religious and spiritual texts. He is concerned about his wife's health problems. They said they do not exercise.

When I gave them my home telephone number, Mrs. Song asked her husband, although he is ten years older than she is, to write it down instead of doing it herself. She delegates any writing to her husband, which seems to be the customary practice. In her age group, most women were not particularly expected to read or write. The division of labor related to gender seems clear.

Reverend and Mrs. Song were quite isolated from the outside world. Most of the elderly Korean informants were busy studying to become citizens of the United States, but Reverend and Mrs. Song said that they hadn't heard anything about it. When I mentioned the citizenship examination, they didn't seem to be concerned about it either. They just thanked me courteously for the news. Because of their advanced age, perhaps they felt that they couldn't really do anything, so they may have taken the passive position, "It's no use worrying about it. Let us not worry about it." Reverend Song may believe that he doesn't need to become a U.S. citizen because of his age. According to some of the informants, some people are exempt from the citizenship examination. The Songs may have been disengaged from most social activities. Or Reverend Song's relaxed, indifferent attitude might be related to his long life and religious experience. When there is a problem, it is better to react with an easy manner and caution.

However, surprisingly, in other matters Reverend Song seemed to be uneasy and much concerned about what others think of them. The phone was disconnected accidentally in the middle of our conversation. When I called back immediately, Reverend Song said the phone company had disconnected it because the conversation that he and I had was too long.

Reverend Song said that he is just waiting to die. He and his wife did not complain of depression, *hwabyung, han,* or *shingyungshayak*. He appears to be ready to accept death as a natural principle. Reverend and Mrs. Song seem to be at the stage of resolution and integrity in life.

WAITING TO DIE NATURALLY

Mrs. Phi is an eighty-eight-year-old widow, a high school graduate, and a very wise and kind intellectual. When she has a ride, she attends a Christian church, using a walker. She lives in a subsidized apartment by herself. She wrote a book about her life in Korea and America. She said that she was really waiting to die. She spoke humbly and sincerely:

> I have one daughter and three sons, and all of them became professionals. My daughters-in-law are all medical doctors. When I get sick and I cannot live alone, I can be sent to a nursing home or a hospital. If I fall down and become unconscious, what can I do when I live alone? My biggest concern is that if I fall down in the kitchen and am unconscious and a fire starts, what do I do?
>
> I saved twenty thousand dollars and gave it to my daughter, a physician in America, for autonomic analgesics, which I heard Mrs. Kennedy used also, in case I suffer from chronic pain. I am still alive because I haven't died or I am not dying yet. That is all.
>
> My grandchildren may call me a ghost because I look like one. The food that I, an old person, cook is unworthy for young people to eat. I am ashamed of myself. I have just become a burden to my children. I can only move around with a broad-based support walker. I live in a most comfortable way. Because no one visits here, I can sleep whenever I like, and I eat a little whenever I like. I live as I want to because nobody sees how I live. To me days and nights are the same. It really doesn't make any difference to me whether it is day, night, evening, weekday, or weekend.
>
> I cannot even pray because I have run out of what to pray for or what to say. I'm not particularly lonely even though I live alone. I wish I could die in my sleep. I live meaninglessly. I have to die before my children die. I am burdensome to them because I cannot help them, but sit and do nothing. Old people should die like a metabolic principle—the old ones should be replaced by new ones. About 99 percent of elderly people are praying to go to heaven, but I do not care to go there. After all,

> heaven is an imaginary place, not a real place for people who are suffering now to escape to.
>
> My husband did not have any human beauty. If one cannot bear to live with one's in-laws and one's husband, as in my case, one has to die. I had suicidal thoughts and was about to attempt to kill myself, but I overcame it for my children. They looked pitiful. I have *hwabyung* still. My husband drank and did not understand what I was going through when I was young.
>
> The things that make me sad are an uncaring attitude, no visits, and no phone calls from my children. When they visit me, I do not want to watch them leaving tired and alone after working hard for me. I regret that I did not do my best, for example, in interpersonal relationships. Sometimes I did not talk to others kindly and gently, although I was feeling tenderly inside myself toward people.

Mrs. Phi uses certain kinds of self-care to feel better, such as whistling, playing a Korean card game (solitaire), playing the harmonica, forgetting unpleasant thoughts, or thinking of pleasant memories of her youth. She is very good at reading, writing, and comprehending Chinese characters. She showed me a wonderful herbal medical prescription in an old Korean traditional medical book written in Chinese. I tried to transcribe the Chinese characters. When she noted that I was writing down the Chinese characters slowly and awkwardly because I hadn't used them for a long time, she took over and wrote them adroitly and beautifully.

Mrs. Phi receives powdered herbs from her daughter in Korea and makes her own all-purpose herbal medicine balls for her high blood pressure, musculoskeletal pains, and eye pain based on the prescription. She said that her herb balls did wonders for her almost all her life. However, recently she noticed a rash on her face and itching in her eyes and skin, and she showed the rash to me. She suspected that it was a symptom of the cumulative side effects of the homemade herb balls. Probably, especially since her kidneys and liver may not work as well as they did when she was younger, toxic wastes may have accumulated in her body. She said, "I occasionally visit my Western physician to ask him to write a death certificate when I die, but nothing else. I heard that you have to have one physician for that purpose in America."

Mrs. Phi wished to die and she described why she is ready to die. She believes that her behavior is not like that of ordinary people, who are full of energy and are aware of what is going on. She feels that she merely exists without the joy of being alive, and neither can she appreciate the wonders and phenomena of the world nor participate actively and independently in it.

She has prepared for her final days. She has tried to avoid burdening her children by giving her daughter money to use in case she has chronic pain. She does not think of allowing herself to live with one of her children regardless of how sick and helpless she will be. She subtly suggested that none of her children will be willing to live with her. She knows that she has to depend on the welfare system. She has helpless feelings about the safety of other people, but not so much for herself because she insists that she has lived long enough and wants to leave this world. She believes that the image of the elderly is ugly. She has low self-esteem and a negative self-concept. Her time concepts are different from those of average people because she does not have to keep time strictly, and her daily activities are quite different from those of fully engaged people. She uses her own flexible, natural, intuitive, and circadian rhythm. She has her own style of cooking, caring for herself, recreation, hobbies, religion, spirituality, and so on.

She has internal conflicts in relating to her children. She needs and likes their support and attention, but she is afraid of troubling them. There really seems to be a time to die peacefully. If so, then it is time for Mrs. Phi to pass away, according to her. Even a couple of years ago, she wanted to listen to philosophy lectures and to do volunteer work. However, this year she has not mentioned these activities, but said, "I am ashamed of myself for being alive still. I wish I could die peacefully. What shall I do to die? When I go to the grocery store with my walker, I feel like people are saying, 'You poor thing. Even an old person such as you is striving to live so hard. Is it not better to drop dead?'" She is very self-conscious and critical of herself and feels unwanted. If she could be given genuine, quality support and attention to develop her potential to the fullest, to be creative and spiritually uplifted, she could enjoy her life again.

However, reality is not so. That is why she wants to die rather than live.

She has been keeping abreast of advances in medicine and has made up her mind to apply advanced analgesics. She reads a Korean newspaper and listens to Korean radio. She understands a little English and occasionally watches American television programs. She said, "I enjoy watching American television programs although I don't understand English. I can sort of guess what's going on."

When I tried to contact her again, all I could discover was that the phone was disconnected. Had she passed away? Was she transferred to a nursing home or her daughter's house because she was unable to care for herself? I felt sad. I missed her kindness, smiles, down-to-earth talks and opinions, wisdom, eccentric lifestyle, and ironic chuckles. She very freely and generously shared her rich experiences of life with me. I hope she is peaceful. Recently, I was able to find out through a mutual acquaintance that she broke her leg and was moved to a nursing home.

Discussion and Conclusion

SOCIODEMOGRAPHIC OBSERVATIONS

Demographically, between the depressives and nondepressives interviewed for this study, there seem to be some differences. Those who were judged to be depressed often had less education, and many were widowed. The two groups did not seem to differ significantly in the number of years they had been in the United States. People between the ages of sixty and seventy seemed to be concerned more about everyday life matters than the Koreans over age eighty. Almost all of the immigrants came to this country to join their children; virtually all initially lived with their adult children, and over time the families have moved apart. More depressives are living separately from their children than nondepressives. More nondepressive (ten) than depressive (four) women live with their husbands. Married informants seem to be better adjusted, less lonely, and tend to be less depressed. More nondepressives are invited to live with their sons than their daughters. More depressives are invited by daughters than sons. In these cases, there may be some problems with a son, which could be a reason to be depressed. Traditionally, parents live with their son or sons. Parents avoid living with a daughter if at all possible. If they do, generally they may be looked down upon because they may be considered as not having a son, or not getting along with the daughter-in-law or son. Sons support parents in the patriarchal tradition while the parents are alive, and venerate them after they have passed away.

Some parents move out of their children's homes. Part of the reason is that the grandchildren whom the grandparents initially cared for have grown up; hence, these elderly immigrants no longer have a reason to live with their children. In part, this reflects American culture, which fosters separate households for the elderly.

Inability to speak English causes most of the informants difficulty in the process of becoming American citizens. Their children or others cannot sit for the citizen examination for the elderly Koreans, as they would interpret for them when they do other things. The elders were most bothered by the problem of obtaining citizenship in order to receive living expenses from the government. Some Korean elders who are illiterate or who think passing the citizen's examination is an unfamiliar, impossible dream just give up on becoming U.S. citizens without any attempts.

Some educated Korean gentlemen and former government officials and professionals seem to be ambivalent about becoming U.S. citizens. It seems to have something to do with loyalty to their mother country. However, it is not easy for them to decide whether to become U.S. citizens because without the government's financial support, it is hard to enjoy independence and freedom, and avoid burdening their children. Most of them are eager to become American citizens. Most of them express that they are Americans and are eager to do volunteer work for the community—especially when their children do not need their assistance—for their health and socialization, sense of well-being, accomplishment, and usefulness.

RECIPROCAL RELATIONS WITH CHILDREN

Although some parents seem to complain initially about their children's lack of care for them, actually they are very protective of their children. Parents do not mind being in a disadvantaged position for the sake of their children.

An elderly woman protected her daughter-in-law to the point of endangering her own health. One of her relatives living nearby found that the elderly woman was critically ill, all alone, and notified her son and his wife to do something about her. This eighty-five-year-old woman did not mention her children's undutiful and unfilial behavior but told her relatives that her son and daughter-in-law did their best for her. She had told her own daughter the same, so her daughter expressed gratitude to her sister-in-law for tender care that she had not even given. After all these events, the elderly woman was offered an opportunity to be cared for by her daughter. She did not accept it because this might devalue what she wanted to credit her son and daughter-in-law with and it might mean a loss of her son's present and future patriarchal rights to her daughter and son-in-law, even though they are the elderly woman's rights now. Only when she did her best to protect her children or other people appropriately could she have peace of mind. She would much rather suffer from physical discomforts or other disadvantages than from the emotional distress, the shame of selfishness, or the guilt of not doing her best as a traditional matriarch, especially since her husband has passed away. If she did otherwise, it would mean to her that she would not be considered a virtuous woman but one with a lack of self-cultivation. Her sense of self is very important with her strong mind and the sense of what to live for, how to act, and how to live according to her standards, beliefs, and practices.

Also, older Koreans and the majority of their adult children have been basically conditioned to the mutual obligation of filial piety. After all, true filial piety is realized with mutual caring between children and parents, although there are times when one generation receives more than they give. The children have been cared for by their parents and the elderly parents are cared for by their children. When we look at this in a continuum, it is a perpetuation of exchange. It is said that among Koreans, there is a longer, overindulged childhood with parental overprotection. The mutual affection, understanding, and care seem to go a long way. An informant said that one of his children who was supported least by him and his wife has been most devoted to them. The child might have been adequately nurtured and reared, although his parents felt that they provided less to him, and he has been grateful for his parents' attention and care. Some children feel indebted to their parents just for being born into this world; some children could be more thankful and responsible. According to the parents, children who are pampered by their parents are not so devoted. They are not aware of the parents' sacrifices. They did not experience difficulties because everything was provided for them.

FILIAL PIETY

Among Koreans, the filial duty of children is an unconditional and genuine responsibility for their parents' health, well-being, satisfaction, and happiness. However, according to observations made by some of the informants and their children, it appears to be conditional and relative based on the parents' degree of sacrifice and fulfillment of their parental duties and responsibilities. Informants who believed that they did not educate their children properly took it as a matter of course when their children did not perform their filial duty by not living near, sharing with, and supporting their parents. A daughter of an informant told her mother that she did not deserve filial veneration because the mother had not given her any money when she was able to. Among Koreans, sons are supposed to be more responsible for caring for their parents, at least in their thoughts, while daughters could be more conditional in supporting their parents. Probably it is because Korea is a patriarchal society. There is a saying that daughters become thieves and *chulgaoein,* which means that they are no longer family members after they are married. After daughters are married, parents and daughters usually do not do much together anymore and when, occasionally, a married daughter visits her parents' home, she is considered greedy if she packs things to take to her husband's home.

When parents and children agree that they are both responsible and devoted, they respect each other. But they perceive mutual caring differently; the two parties seem to have conflicts in their relationships.

Some informants proudly said that their children support them very well because the informants did everything possible for their children first. However, the pattern of filial duty cannot be generalized. To some children, filial piety can be unconditional. Devotion is demonstrated splendidly regardless of the quality of parental care when children understand the difficult circumstances their parents went through, or simply because of the fact that their parents bore them. It is very important to have the opportunity to share life experiences between parents and children. The morality of the family and the self-interest of the caregiver (Mackenzie and Holroyd, 1995; Ngan and Cheng, 1992) and social conditions (Finch, 1989) are delicately intertwined in a caring family. Most of the informants and their children live by the principle of filial piety, which is rooted in Korean and Confucian tradition.

CHANGES IN GENDER ROLES

Some informants had a hard time tolerating nontraditional gender roles in men. Nontraditional distributions of labor are beginning to appear in Korean immigrant families. The informants' sons cook or do dishes. It is very hard for elderly Korean parents to face and accept this. In this case, some elders move out or return to Korea, so that they don't have to see and suffer from "ugly and unacceptable" scenes.

However, some of the informants willingly compromise to help adult children by taking nontraditional gender roles themselves. For example, a father-in-law helps his daughter-in-law wash the dishes or set the table. One daughter-in-law praised this helpful behavior enough to write a poem about it and have it published in a church newsletter.

CREATING HARMONY WITH CHILDREN

A reason for the tendency to reminisce about the past instead of talking about current affairs is to make peace and create harmony by understanding the children's situations instead of making things more complicated by criticizing them. There is a Korean saying, "If you accept all things both fair and ugly about others and your environment, everything will be harmonious and peaceful and loving." Koreans are reluctant to make any negative comments about or to their children because it is not considered virtuous and cultivated. Some Korean elders might say, "How pitiful it is to speak ill of our own children or even of other children!" Also, children should not speak ill of their parents under any circumstances, although they can be corrected kindly about their wrong behaviors. Their guiding principle is, if children or others need to be reprimanded, do so directly or through some other close, respected elder.

PAST TRAUMAS

The Korean elders talked about their painful pasts more than the conditions of their current lives. There are several possible reasons for this phenomenon. Some of them are better off in America than they were in Korea. If they have problems, they want to solve them by themselves quietly as often as possible. The majority of the informants believe that it is ugly to speak ill of their loved ones and others. Also, they believe that it may risk their integrity and reputation, and cause interpersonal problems.

Without history there is no present or future. Perhaps the elders' past consists only of memories of their hardships and now they are in the stage of reminiscence and it surpasses problems faced here and now.

Many elders have kept their traumas inside too long, including the experiences of deaths of family members, poverty, their "blood, sweat, and tears" efforts to survive the oppression and atrocities of the Japanese occupation, and the cruelty of the Korean War. Women had to find means of survival since men were out of regular work during the crises. They may be suffering from delayed post-traumatic stress disorder from the cruelest experiences. Some informants were distressed by recurrent painful recollections of events, illusions, and intense psychological distress at exposure to the events that symbolize or resemble an aspect of the traumatic event. These included: anniversaries, a restricted range of affect such as being unable to have spontaneous loving feelings toward persons who betrayed, rejected, or abused them, feelings of detachment or estrangement from others, difficulty falling or staying asleep, irritability, or outbursts of anger as described in the DSM-III-R (American Psychiatric Association, 1987).

THE NEED TO RECIPROCATE

Friendship plays an important role in meeting elderly Korean immigrants' needs, especially when family members are not able to assist them. Friends can be substitutes for family members. One of the drawbacks can be the thoughts and feelings of indebtedness of the recipient when exchanges between friends are not balanced. Some of the informants are reluctant to receive assistance even when they are in need. As soon as they appreciate others' kindness, they start to worry about repayment, saying, "How can I pay back what I owe to everybody in this apartment building?" One of the informants invited all the residents to a luncheon party in her apartment building on a Saturday afternoon; she spent close to one thousand dollars, which had been sent by her son for her eightieth birthday. The money was intended to be used for airfare to visit him in Korea. Her daughter and niece bought huge quantities of prepared food from a Korean market, and they cooked more dishes themselves. A Korean woman in the same apartment building told me that this woman was very indebted to almost everybody in the apartment complex and her family members should show their gratitude somehow to the apartment residents. There are certain expectations for exchange. It is good to reciprocate, but there seems to be social pressure for it even before one is ready.

THE STRUGGLE FOR HARMONY THROUGH INDEPENDENCE

Even if elderly Koreans have difficult problems, they don't want to make the situation worse by complaining, or they may think that nobody will understand and nothing can be done. They were used to solving their own problems when they were young and energetic, but now the situation has changed. They are no longer young and energetic. They have to make sociocultural adjustments, directly and indirectly. Often they are not familiar with ways to meet their basic needs in America. They have to depend on others for most of their needs. Still, some Korean elders might think that as they overcame tribulations in the past, they shall solve their current problems also, and if not, they just have to bear them.

Korean elders tend to choose the options that could bring them peace of mind. They may choose to work physically or do away with things to avoid bothering others. That way they don't have to be concerned about what others think of them. They know that people will be glad to do things for them, at least sometimes, but they usually decline the offer so as not to burden them and, in turn, they are not burdened emotionally. Koreans are familiar with the sayings: "Be glad of drinking water and eating herbs and vegetables instead of being greedy with a gourmet," and "I can live without that. Not having that won't kill me. Don't kill yourself to get me that!"

In particular, those who were very poor and oppressed in Korea seem to appreciate their present conditions in America, such as having food and housing from their children or from the government. However, they still need to handle their basic needs in the unfamiliar, foreign maze of the psychosocially and culturally different American society. Some of them have developed a support network.

A Korean elder whom I have known for fifteen years came to America to assist her daughter who was expecting a child and, subsequently, she cared for her three granddaughters. She later moved out of her daughter's house to her subsidized apartment. Some of her reasons for moving out were that her granddaughters were grown up, she felt unappreciated by her granddaughters, her son-in-law did not want her in his house any longer, and her own daughter subtly wished her mother would move out so that they could enjoy their nuclear family lifestyle. The whole family is busy going to work or school.

When this woman broke her leg, her granddaughter took her to the clinic for a follow-up appointment since her daughter had to work in her own take-out restaurant all day and the woman had removed her son-in-law from her support network. It seemed that he was always busy and did not really care about his mother-in-law. This grandmother was not pleased that her granddaughter had to accompany her, because her granddaughter, a junior in high school, was too young and too inexperienced to take that kind of responsibility. Then she called her niece for her next clinic visit. Again, the grandmother was not satisfied. She felt that surgery should be performed because a bone was "sticking out," but her niece went along with the physician's nonsurgical treatment regimen. For her next clinical visit, she decided to hire a Korean who could speak English, drive, and had accompanied other residents in her apartment building. No resident helper asks for a fee for this service, but the helper is usually given twenty to thirty dollars, with the customary saying, "You have worked very hard. Please, just buy lunch for yourself with this money although it is not much." The assistance gives the helper something to do as well as a sense of helping others. The woman's daughter said that they called the community service center but they charged for their services.

DOES FATALISM STOP PEOPLE FROM HELPING THEMSELVES?

The fatalism of elderly Korean immigrants has empowered them to endure, persevere, and overcome their destiny by accepting their fate or their troubles. This contrasts with the popular belief that fatalism entraps people with thoughts that they cannot change anything because of the fate with which they were born. However, there are nearly always alternatives or other opportunities when adversity is unavoidable. Koreans at least recognize their sincere effort to do their best. Because they believe that fate is predestined, they are motivated to do their best, to appreciate or endure the fulfillment of duty and responsibility, to participate and achieve the goals of nature and the universe, and even to transcend their fate. Positively and actively accepting fate is a process of revitalization, reenergization, renewal, and re-creation of a new direction. Each individual's contribution is a unique mission. Nobody has exactly the same fate. Fate is like important missionary work, and it calls for doing one's best. Someone who does not believe in fate might neglect another's expectation and be ostracized. For example, one of the Korean elders in this study had become a young widow with young children, forced to live in poverty. If she did not have a sense of fate about her unexpected widowhood, the woman might have abandoned her children and her duty as set by nature and Korean society. After all, based on the informants' narratives, Koreans may believe in fatalism, which is defined as "a doctrine that events are fixed in advance for all time in such a manner that human beings are powerless to change them" (*Webster's New Collegiate Dictionary,* 1979). Even if someone believes in the definition of fate as stated in Webster's dictionary, fate may confine or limit an aspect of life, but almost all other avenues will be open. If we go back to the widow, she had unlimited resources and opportunities to make her situation better and to empower herself, her children, and even her neighbors. She could motivate herself instead of succumbing to disappointment. The Korean elders survived with one another's support in networks and expanded their sources of income with projects such as sewing, hoeing, peddling, and running small or even big businesses during and after the Korean War. There are sayings in Korea: "If you really, sincerely, and earnestly wish for something worthwhile and do your best, heaven will be impressed with you and will help you to achieve it," or "A mother's earnest and sincere wish for her children will move even a huge mountain." It seems that fate is accompanied by unlimited possibilities and positive forces that can turn around adversity. "Crises are opportunities."

KOREANS AND CHONG

There seem to be two groups of informants. One group had hardships in the past and now has a satisfactory life, and the other group had hardships in the past and is still having hardships. The latter seems to suffer from lack of *chong,* that is, an ability to share and receive spontaneous, holistic understanding, empathy, sympathy, warmth, and care from others. Frequently, foreign residents in Korea describe *chong* as an impressive, unique experience. *Chong* is a characteristic of Koreans, and it is expressed tangibly and intangibly, even when meeting someone for the first time, in daily life. Koreans address one another with kinship terms even if they are strangers. For example, if a person resembles your mother in her feelings toward you, her appearance, or her age, then you would call her "mother," and so on. A person can be called grandfather, grandmother, father, mother, uncle, aunt, brother, or sister according to gender, age, role, degree of informality, and comfort level in addressing someone informally. One may call someone by a professional title such as "teacher," even if the person is not a real teacher, if one respects the person and would like to relate to them in terms of that role.

However, this compassionate behavior appears to diminish gradually as an individualistic society emerges; most Korean informants long for *chong,* especially as they get old and increasingly desire support. Essentially, those who are deprived of *chong* suffer from Korean illness or depression. Thus, *chong* can heal people.

When things are going well, Korean elders tend to attribute it primarily to their children and when they are not, the elders still attribute it to their children. Some of them might blame their ancestors and/or fate as well. There is a saying among certain people in Korea that when things go wrong, ancestors are to blame. *Chong* is the vital energy—the psychosocial, spiritual, biological, ethical, moral, and existential force of compassion—circulating among people to distribute the essences of life, such as family care, food, clothes, money, health care, and even leisure activities. Most of the Koreans pour out *chong* to their children first and later expect to receive *chong* from them, although these days they say, "We should not expect to receive anything from children." *Chong* is needed in old age more than at any other time. *Chong* is expected from their children, although most of them receive financial assistance from the government.

When all members of a family emanate *chong* among themselves as expected, harmony, peace, mutual respect, dignity, and a sense of well-being are created. When a balance of *chong* is not created—for example, when one expresses *chong* to someone and the other does not return it—a person may experience rejection, betrayal, indifference, or distress. This kind of condition (negative feelings and thoughts) may develop into depression, *han*, *hwabyung*, and/or *shingyungshayak*. In particular, people who tend to emanate *chong* without any expectation of receiving it from others are considered virtuous, respected, and dignified persons. These kinds of people are called transcended people and they enjoy immense peace, harmony, and health.

Some behavioral examples of *chong* include visiting with a lonely old mother, father, or someone in the community, being kind and doing something together; listening attentively to someone who needs to be heard; understanding someone who needs to be understood; supporting someone in need of support. Other examples: feeding the hungry; sheltering someone who needs housing; interpreting; giving a ride to someone or taking them to a clinic; teaching someone how to become a citizen of the United States; calming the fears of someone who is afraid to die alone or to live alone or go to a nursing home; seeking solutions together; helping someone go to the grocery store; respecting each other as dignified human beings; asking if anything can be done; doing or giving something without expecting anything in return. Also, *chong* is accepting something thoughtful with ethical and moral considerations in mind, such as a helping hand offered by the elderly.

However, *chong* is different from fulfilling an obligation, because *chong* means doing something good for others or readily expressing something worthwhile with compassion and spontaneity. For Korean elders, *chong* can be very therapeutic for both the receiver and the giver. It works as an essence and energizer for life, and as medicine for healing.

Koreans characterize volatile emotions, such as rage or frustration, as dangerous, bringing harm to themselves and others. That is why people are warned to govern themselves with cultivation and equanimity, with sayings such as "Get angry slowly," or "If you can govern yourself, you can govern the whole world." Also, Koreans describe illnesses or emotions, especially negative ones such as anger, as tangible, structural, patterned, and material. They said things such as, "The fire and blood were pushed up," or "Anger was pushed to the stomach and chest." Fire is described as boiling heat and is a symbol of a destructive force that is capable of destroying mental and physical health, and interpersonal and psychosocial functions. The displaced emotion is expressed as a physical symptom. Negative emotions may be felt as lumps through a somatization process. Such lumps are usually intangible by laboratory test or physical palpation, although they cause physical discomfort. Storytelling and sharing may bring relief of the distress when it is channeled through the support of loved, active listeners with *chong* by using the idioms of *han, hwabyung,* or other illnesses.

For some parents and children, living in separate households relieves stress and depression as well as illnesses. *Life Style and Value System of the Aged in Korea,* compiled and published by Korea Survey (Korea Survey Gallup Polls, 1990), suggested that separate households for the elderly are increasing, although the majority live with their children in Korea. Those who identified themselves or were identified by DIS-III as nondepressives have self-confidence, a positive personality, and look forward to their future. They have trusting relationships with their children and others. They are able to appreciate family life. They have flexibility in decision making for themselves. For example, usually they can live with the family or alone in an apartment according to their wishes, or are supported by their children. Also, they enjoy the health, the freedom, and the independence to make decisions and carry out their own plans, such as visiting Korea. They appreciate their happy situations, which makes them even more contented.

Some informants, who claim that they have neither depression nor illnesses such as *hwabyung,* claimed that those who complain of depression or Korean illnesses are immature, uncultivated persons or cowards, regardless of the magnitude of hardships and tribulations that the depressives experienced. The people who criticized did not care what kinds of problems the depressives had or what kinds of attitudes, character, or personalities they possessed.

KOREAN POPULAR ILLNESSES

Older Korean immigrants work through the lay diagnoses of *hwabyung* and other illnesses for their health by telling the stories of their distress to outsiders who have no conflict of interest with them or with their family. Nineteen out of twenty-one of those who had major depression mentioned one or more Korean popular illnesses, as shown in the following table.

Occurrence of Korean Popular Illnesses

(N = 21; 3 men and 18 women with major depression)

Illness	Men	Women
Hwabyung	1	10
Shingyungshayak	1	2
Hwabyung and *Shingyungshayak*	0	2
Han, Hwabyung, and *Shingyungshayak*	0	2
Han and *Hwabyung*	0	1
No Korean Popular Illnesses	1	1
Total	3	18

Mrs. Lee, a Korean elder, could not distinguish whether the pains she felt were physical or mental. She added that when she had that sort of pain, she didn't want to do anything at all. There seem to be no physical, emotional, psychosocial, or spiritual pains in extremely unpleasant situations, such as a grandson's betrayal or a daughter-in-law's nagging, but instead a holistic pain. Physical pain can be an expression of emotional pain, emotional pain can express spiritual pain, and all kinds of pain are related and become holistic. It is the older Koreans' belief that this kind of total pain could cause ailments such as cardiac disease. I call it holistic pain since I have not yet found a better name. Before they leave this world, Korean elders seem to have the urge to resolve their pain. They wish to share with people who are willing to listen to them in order to come to terms with the true meaning of their pain. Then they can die peacefully with dignity and respect.

HOLISM: EXPRESSIONS OF EMOTIONAL DISTRESS IN PHYSICAL TERMS

The phenomena of psychologization and somatization among Chinese and Americans were compared, and the results suggest that the Chinese tend to somatize more than the Americans, while Americans tend to psychologize more than the Chinese (Kleinman, 1980: 174). It might be interesting to explore how elderly Korean immigrants deal with and resolve this issue.

Koreans believe that emotional distress should be "digested" in the body, not expressed verbally. When hurt feelings are not properly digested, or when an initial shock is felt, they tend to say things such as, "The organs and intestines are burning!" Some cannot digest at all due to fire or lack of self-cultivation.

Jae Guan Lee (1997: 204) stated: "From time to time, I remember the pain of my chest being torn out when I was watching my wife crying as she was holding our blood-stained dead son." He described his emotional state in terms of physically felt pain. Reverend Yil Do Choi (1995) confessed in his autobiography that he felt pains, as though his chest was torn out, as he was being insulted and rejected by a shelter manager who belonged to a different denomination, when Reverend Choi tried to get a needy person a temporary shelter.

Sometimes it is very difficult to distinguish whether someone is complaining of an actual physical symptom or of emotional distress, for example, "My vigor [bone marrow and blood] has been all dried up!" or "My eyes are always wet due to inner fire." These expressions are used by people who feel exhausted physically and mentally, especially in old age. It is difficult to say whether they are related to the mind or the body. Both influence each other by intra- and interpersonal, social, environmental, and cosmological factors. When a person is severely distressed the mind and body are both damaged, although it may not be literally to the degree that they claim. Wan-Suh Park (1995), a writer, described in her autobiography: "The being torn out was not my mind. But it was like a part of my body, so that I examined my body here and there to find where it was being torn out in a chaotic, bewildering manner," when she was remorseful. People who question their own ethical and moral behaviors and conclude that they are not up to par are tortured by feelings of guilt and shame. They could be verbalized, for example, as "It hurts my chest."

One of our informants, Mr. Moon, stated that when he was verbally insulted by his "untamed" daughter, it was both emotionally and physically agonizing. He was in such a fury that he had to leave her immediately and go to an emergency room because he was having chest pains. Mr. Moon mentioned that he has *hwabyung,* which could cause death. The emotional distress is intense, and it seems to involve both the physical and the emotional. Mr. Moon's case is a typical example of *hwabyung* among Koreans.

When emotional distress is intensified and prolonged, pathophysiological changes will take place. There seems to be no such thing as a purely emotional or physical reaction. The more the emotional state is intensified, the more the physical health loses its equilibrium. The more severe the emotional distress or threat, the more severe will be the physical threat or injury.

In mild to moderate degrees of psychological and somatic realization, there seem to be no visible physical signs and symptoms, although people describe their distress in somatic terms. In the mild to moderate emotional state with a great deal of physically felt distress, there may be some real hormonal and chemical changes, although they are not manifested grossly, objectively, or visibly. It might be entirely up to the individual's capacity to adapt to stress. In any case, discussion of biochemical and physiological changes are beyond the scope of this book.

Each individual seems to manifest symptoms differently. Some may stay at the emotional level and some may suffer from both emotional and physical symptoms. It might have a great deal to do with personality, level of cultivation, and the kind and degree of adaptation to a distressing condition or situation. Usually, Koreans express themselves as "digesting" or "killing unreasonably angry self" internally and quietly so that nobody will notice it. It is common to use derogatory or self-blaming expressions even though they have not done anything terrible.

The viability of human life is usually described in terms of physiological function and integrity. It seems easier to describe life in terms of the body than the mind and emotion. Generally, people think the body is tangible and concrete while the mind is abstract and intangible. When emotional shock is severe, people seem to perceive and express it as though the body has lost physical integrity. Among Korean elders, it is understood that anger particularly injures the liver according to traditional Korean medical understanding. Everybody understands life-threatening physical danger, but people infrequently speak in terms of life-threatening emotional danger. In Korean society, also, expressing drudgery, lack of enthusiasm, depressed mood, emotional disability, psychosocial maladjustment, or psychiatric illness is discouraged. Thus, Koreans use pathophysiological idioms to express emotional pain and physiological malfunction. When they do that, people understand it readily. Highly cultivated, religious, spiritual, and wise persons might have a better chance of maintaining mind-body integrity.

Koreans may use different, indirect methods of psychologization. I tend to think that they psychologize and somatize simultaneously, which is different from the previous emphasis on somatization only. Koreans seem to synthesize and synergize the two. However, do elderly Korean people psychologize less than others do? They tend to heal themselves through holistic psychologization-somatization. Their ideal resolution is to digest and regulate distress internally through the process of understanding, interpretation, analysis, synthesis, acceptance, spirituality, and transcendence of emotional-physical problems caused by internal and external factors.

When mind and emotion are distressed, the informants seem to believe that the mind and emotion dwell inside the body and the organs. Distress makes all the vital internal organs seem chaotic, depleted or overly full, shrunken, or swollen. In extremely shocking or stressful situations, the injured mind decays and destroys internal organs and paralyzes the whole person. Since the condition is physical, psychological, and internalized, the informants use physical remedies and mental therapies. Some examples of physical remedies are: various physical exercises including breathing exercises, acupressure, acupuncture, and diet therapies for functional and structural restoration as a vital energy aid in the natural environment. Some examples of mental therapies are: seeking alternative problem-solving strategies, catharsis with a confidant, diversion, changing thinking patterns to new directions, and self-cultivation. Elderly Korean immigrants believe that problems should be internalized; otherwise they will grow out of proportion and will be very difficult to handle, causing chaotic interpersonal relationships. Caring for one's own mind-body will resolve the mind-body injury.

Elderly Korean immigrants seem to respond to violence and suffering by blaming themselves, although, at the beginning, they sometimes appear to blame others who made them suffer. They direct these responses to themselves and digest the injuries and hurt by themselves.

Sooshin, which in Korean literally means body training, is better known as a form of self-cultivation. However, *sooshin* involves both mind and body. This phenomenon supports the coexistence of psychologization and somatization. They represent mind-body connections, although emotional distress could be emphasized more than bodily injury or vice versa (psychologization versus somatization).

Hwabyung seems to be combined with anger, anxiety, and depression. *Hwabyung* is the typical example of the holistic representation of distress and a syndrome of biopsychological and sociocultural factors. Acute *hwabyung* indicates an extremely critical psychological and physical condition requiring immediate attention with medical, psychosocial, and interpersonal support.

As soon as people share their stories of *hwabyung, han,* or *shingyungshayak,* an explanatory model and semantic network of their illness is provided, and care is started based on the cause, diagnosis, symptomatology, treatment regimen, and predicted efficacy. The value of culture-specific illnesses is their role in therapeutic processes. These narratives consist of all the processes.

THE BLESSINGS OF KOREAN POPULAR ILLNESSES

When Korean elders are distressed by events such as language difficulties and conflicts with children, they embody them in the mind, emotions, and soul. If the mind, emotions, and soul are distressed and injured, then sometimes the injured mind, emotions, and soul will cause various ailments in the body, such as heart disease, indigestion, etc. Most elderly Koreans tend to explain causes of mental and physical diseases in terms of cosmological, natural, psychosocial, ethical, and moral phenomena, not just biologically based reasoning.

Hwabyung, as a sufferer-oriented explanatory model, aids the sufferer and health care providers, and it has efficacy. The etiology, symptoms, diagnosis, and related self-care have been orchestrated harmoniously in terms of narrative behaviors and simultaneous catharsis, insight, and continuous self-cultivation. *Hwabyung* as well as *han* and *shingyungshayak* give people the opportunity to look at themselves and review their lifestyles, personalities, and psychosocial behaviors holistically, in order to understand and evaluate themselves and improve their lifestyles more harmoniously by regulating their judgments, emotions, and behaviors. By meditation and self-cultivation, they try to transcend the ordinary emotions of anger, frustration, and stress in order to achieve a healthy, peaceful, and harmonious mental and physical condition.

SELF-CARE

Korean elders use certain social interactions as a method for feeling better. Humor is used to treat stress and manage illnesses. The use of humor with jokes, books, and music can reduce pain and enhance joy. It allows them to release anger in a socially acceptable way, establish and ease relationships, and relieve anxiety. Humor is commonly acknowledged by Korean elders as therapeutic in creating good feelings. They are consoled and inspired by themselves and the encouragement of others. Humor helps us to share, communicate, and to have esprit de corps.

Direct, aggressive emotional catharsis has been discouraged in Korean elders because they were taught not to become angry but to show dignity and remain undisturbed. However, some elders admitted that they were hysterical with their children and were only waiting for death (Pang, 1996). Some informants seem to stay chronically depressed and never seem to fully resolve it. They regulate their difficult feelings by accepting some feelings and giving up others to maintain harmony with self and others in combination with physical movements such as taking a walk. Actually, this is a holistic, therapeutic practice involving emotional, cognitive, spiritual, and physical activities. An example of an environmental change made by Korean elders was moving out to live away from their children and grandchildren, to avoid conflicts with them and to increase mutual comfort. Some of the informants say that living away from their children is like living in heaven, and the few who strongly believe that parents and adult children should live together say it is like living in hell. Some of the examples of phrases used in the Korean elders' therapeutic processes are: "Don't get angry quickly! Take it easy! Know yourself. Be open and flexible with oneself and others."

RESOLVING DEPRESSION

Factors that act as buffers against depression for elderly Koreans seem to be maturity, good health, resilience, being over age eighty, being married, living with children, and having religious and spiritual faith. They can be considered spiritually enlightened. They have easygoing, accepting personalities and cultivated characters so that they do not worry unnecessarily. Education seems to be influential in preventing depression. The more educated are better able to adapt. The educated informants seem to rationalize and act to avoid worries or distress, and they are not drawn into certain circumstances, so they do not worry or grieve. One highly educated elderly professional couple eulogized and glorified their deceased son as a wonderful public servant who dedicated himself to his country. This consoled them at the same time and, thus, they were not in distress.

The majority of the immigrants seem to benefit holistically from spiritual and religious self-care. A Korean gentleman who went to church, believed in a shaman's healing practices, and also saw a psychiatrist, now neither participates in the Korean immigrant church nor sees a psychiatrist. He manages his life and health with self-care including regulated daily activities: seeing friends, shopping by bus, cooking health foods, taking a Korean tonic medicine, taking a walk, reading the newspaper, listening to music, reminiscing, playing hide and seek by himself, and writing his autobiography to share with his children, relatives, friends, and others. He uses a pluralistic medical system including Korean traditional medicine and vitamins. He is confident and proud of his holistic self-care and his youthful health. He sometimes says, "I do not look like an eighty-year-old man. I have rosy cheeks and I dye my hair black."

SPIRITUAL AWARENESS

Self-cultivation has been explained in relation to Confucianism, but these days a significant number of informants seem to be saved and cultivated by Christianity, since most of them, like Mrs. Yong, go to a Christian church and have Christian faith. Maturity seems to be possible only through experiencing hardships. Most of the informants who suffered relate to themselves and others with peace and love. Buddhism is also used in a similar way. As shown in Mrs. You's case, antagonistic and hostile relationships were diverted into peaceful ones through spiritual insight in combination with cognitive change, not fixation. The religious effects could be thought of as syncreticism because Korea is a multireligious country. Confucianism, Buddhism, and shamanism are understood by everybody, especially the elderly immigrants.

Those informants who said they had religious faith (mostly Christians) seem to have peace of mind. Most of the informants, whether or not they professed a religion, somehow resolved their emotional conflicts and distress. Some of them attributed it to religion, God, Jesus, fate, Buddha, self, maturity, cultivation, personality, the mind, *ch'enyom*, intellect, work, exercises, or a combination of these things. The common element seems to have something to do with the self, the will, and the mind, including personality and attitude toward life, and spiritual orientation. Most of them seem to be saying life was hard but it was worthwhile, meaningful, and made sense because they were devoted to finding the meaning of agony and found it according to their own interpretations of life experiences. Especially important was the thought that they worked hard for the next generation, and ultimately for society, so that finally, they could experience peace.

Religion and personal attributes such as an adaptable character and personality, hobbies, and interpersonal support including a confidant are wonderful resources for the healthy and joyful person. But having only one source, such as a confidant, might not be sufficient for harmonious living, as Murphy stated (1982).

The Koreans experienced various kinds of hardships, especially interpersonal conflicts such as spousal abuse or loss of loved ones. By reminiscing and narrating *(nucduri),* they were earnestly seeking the reason for and meaning of hardships. They usually found that religion and spirituality strengthened them with insight and cultivation. They were ready to accept these spiritual processes and serve themselves and others with love and peace. Some informants realized retrospectively that what they endured was worthwhile and rewarded them with dignity, honor, respect, and esteem, especially from their children. Eventually the informants appeared to solve their problems individually or collectively through their support networks and resources.

Generally, the Korean informants, influenced by their animistic cultural beliefs, renew and revitalize themselves by interacting, reflecting, projecting, and casting away worries, conflicts, and distress by submerging themselves in nature and supernatural powers, for example, God, Buddha, or other gods embodied in the moon, sun, stars, big trees and big rocks, and so on.

Mature and cultivated people claim that *sang byung* (creating illnesses unnecessarily due to a lack of broad understanding of human nature and wisdom) could be prevented if people are generous, flexible, and insightful in thinking and action. Also, they believe that if one is kind to others, others will be kind in return, and they practice appropriately. Trusting God has been effective, according to the testimonies of the majority of the informants. Those who believe in Buddhism explain that believing in self is believing in a spiritual religious being. They encourage people to believe in what they think is right.

Some of the Korean elders use the term *ch'enyom* as wise thinking in dealing with self and others for a harmonious and peaceful community. These people might have insight into mental maturity and peacefulness. They are mature with a logical, broad, open, deep understanding, and a foresighted, wise, cultivated, stable, reasonable, unhurried, tolerant, patient, and uplifted soul. They emanate dignity and draw dignity. These people, who might have had a *hwabyung*-like illness already without realizing it, may have fewer, the same, or even more hardships than those who currently express *han, hwabyung,* or *shingyungshayak.*

Those who admit suffering from *han, hwabyung,* or *shingyung-shayak* might be referred to as late bloomers, according to the informants, in transcending emotional and spiritual agony, conflicts, distress, and suffering. Nevertheless, the Korean informants, depressives or nondepressives, have been suffering, knowingly or unknowingly, from at least one Korean popular illness in various degrees when considering the hardships they have had in America as immigrants and in Korea when they were poor and oppressed. To free themselves from the shackles of misery and mortification, the Korean elders used key idioms such as *han, hwabyung,* or *shing-yungshayak* to share the burdens with people and spiritual supernatural beings for understanding, cleansing, sympathy and communion in bliss, harmony, peace, and pride. They have endured and realized the true meaning of the enormous sufferings they went through as the finale of a great tragedy that becomes a comedy, so that they can laugh aloud and transcend the experience and let others see their lifelong masterpiece and triumph. That is their victory!

Jong-ho Yu (1997: 90) writes about Chung-in Su's novel: "Perceiving the limits of dark, weak and guilty elements of the human soul does not always lead to pessimism. A dark perspective sometimes helps us realize the need for humor and tolerance." A good example of this statement is that the elderly Koreans are feeling, living, and having good relationships with themselves and others. They have become insightful, strengthened, and matured to appreciate the meanings of their colorful lives through their destined odyssey.

Korean elders have private, personal, and public expressions of depression and Korean popular illnesses. There seem to be several reasons for the personal side. In order not to bother family and oneself by taking a sick role (to be natural and "normal"), not to be considered a mental, spiritual, and existential weakling, to maintain dignity and not to be stigmatized, Koreans would say *nae sak ahn hada* (not showing inner colors or mood to others). This means that one does not share or publicize something going on inside. It could be a stigmatized illness, secrets, inner conflicts, or worries. A positive response to publicizing an illness could be obtaining support, empathy, and sympathy. Some adverse responses would be rejection or alienation from some people. One of the informants did not share her depressed mood for fear of losing her housekeeping work. Korean elders tend to be less inhibited and talk more freely than when they were young, now that they feel safe to talk about their thoughts and feelings.

Those who have endured severe abuse and loss seem to appreciate the real meaning of life through faith in what they believe. They have come to their own terms for the meaning of hardships that they accepted as fate and endured nobly, dutifully, and responsibly.

Korean elders are distressed by depressive experiences caused by the problems and changes of interpersonal and financial support, and the spiritual aspect of self relating to aging and health problems. Korean elders primarily conceptualized depression with moral and spiritual, psychosocial, and cultural origins instead of only biological explanations. The oldest elders, usually over eighty, who do not have to deal with many problems of everyday life and interpersonal relationships, say that their Korean illnesses are resolved.

In a way, elderly Korean immigrants were normal depressives. They were depressed if they were poor and could not educate their children. They worked all the time. When the people they trusted without doubt and reservation rejected them, they endured it silently. They did not have time to be sick and naturally they were neither hospitalized nor took antidepressants. When they were economically better off and had restored their interpersonal relationships, they would be in better health.

The ways Korean elders use to become whole, meaningful, and spiritual beings are changing thoughts and moods, changing decision making from negative to positive directions, being patient, and being less demanding, more understanding and yielding instead of confronting or fighting for personal gains and rights. The informants use *ch'enyom,* as they say colloquially, "I have to kill myself, give in or give up my desire and need in order to yield for others. That's the best way and the peaceful way." That way they are dignified and respected, and their children and others tend to be willing to support them. However, receiving support from others is not their primary concern but it could be serendipitous. When they or others deviate from moral standards or expectations, elderly Koreans may feel sad, disappointed, or depressed but try not to express these emotions. They do not readily let others know their grudges or complaints because they believe it is best to maintain peace or at least to continue the status quo out of acceptance, true understanding, and self-cultivation, not out of repression and suppression.

Also, others try not to remind family and friends of events in their painful, tragic past. However, when people listen with empathic ears, it is appreciated and becomes therapeutic.

Most Koreans seem to turn their attention toward themselves only when their children and other family members' needs and wishes have been met. If their situation allows, they spend more time with their friends. They go for sightseeing trips, so-called filial tourism, which is supposed to be supported by the children as part of their repayment to their parents for their sacrifices, for bringing the children into this world, rearing, and educating them. In reality, while some children pay for the sightseeing trips, some of the elders pay for them themselves.

Some frail elderly women live by themselves most of the time. They don't see many friends and they don't keep track of time accurately because they live pretty much by their own schedule, biological clock, and lifestyle. These elders expressed that they are really comfortable in a way. Nobody demands anything from them and they live as they like. They sleep when they like, eating when and what they like. In a sense, however, there is too much freedom and they do not spend time meaningfully. The body-mind is not well coordinated. They want to do many useful activities but they cannot. One of the informants said that she really wishes to die because her time has come, but not out of depression or suicidal thoughts. She feels it is simply time for her to go. Elders wish that they could go to the other world when they want to.

Traditionally oriented elderly Koreans tend not to talk openly with their children in America about their futures, life as elderly persons, and death. They doubt that they would ever have a chance to do that because it is such a delicate, taboo subject. It is considered unnatural to discuss it. Although some parents and children make separate preparations for the funeral by selecting clothes to wear to the funeral or setting aside money, they don't talk about it or do those things together. In some cases, doing so might only cause an uncomfortable, emotionally stressful experience for parents and children.

Elderly parents and their children seem to live day by day with a belief or trust that it is all set and understood between them by tradition, sometimes with *yshim chunshim* (filial piety, insight, and intuition without actual talking). Taoism teaches that doing nothing is better than overdoing. Nature will take care of things, including people, when the time comes. Just being and letting nature take care of itself would be more harmonious and peaceful, even more satisfying, than doing. Birth and life occur naturally, so why not death?

One Korean elder expressed fear of the process of dying, but not fear of death itself. Thus, this elder wished that death would come painlessly and quickly. One informant showed curiosity about death.

Korean elders would say *maum merk da* ("I eat my mind")—to be determined, to make up one's mind, or to make body and mind become one. Or they would say *mert yt gae sal da* (to be happy, not depressed, to live fully and meaningfully with style and vision)—to live by sharing with, caring for, and loving others. And in that way they bring vitality and harmony into their lives.

In a broad sense, the majority of the elderly Koreans who were identified as having major depression by DSM-III criteria seem like nondepressives in reality. They too function fully in the family. They neither have taken antidepressants nor have been hospitalized. These Koreans have been convinced by their life experiences that a strongly cultivated individual mind, soul, and will create holistic harmony and health.

According to Korean philosophy, the human will is the origin of nature, harmony, health, and life itself. Mind, soul, will, and body are one in nature, all related as a whole. This holistic human being initiates and influences how one thinks, behaves, and what one generates, such as harmony.

Glossary of Selected Terms

(Note: Glossary terms are in the following order: Western spelling, Korean, Chinese, and interpretation in English.)

badook 바둑: A board game of strategy played with black and white smooth, round, flat stones.

baree up da 발이 없다 (not having "feet"): Having no transportation or ride.

bok i up neun saram i da 복이 없는 사람이다: A person who believes that he or she is not blessed with happiness as he or she deserves or wishes to be.

ch'enyom 체념 諦念: Accepting and resolving distress with an understanding of the inevitable.

chong 정 情: Holistic behaviors that originate, create, and emanate spontaneously and truly compassionate relationships.

chulgaoein 출가외인 出嫁外人: A married daughter is considered no longer a member of her own family when she is married. She becomes an official member of her husband's household. The close relationship with her birth family no longer exists after marriage. Her brother's wife becomes a formal member of her birth family.

chun sang yon boon 천생연분 天生緣分: A perfect marriage is matched, blessed, and destined in heaven with perfect harmony. This expression is used for a man and woman who are in a perfect, harmonious relationship.

gasm ari 가슴아리: Chest illness.

ge 계 契: Collection of a mutual trust fund. Usually, once a month people have meetings for *ge,* perhaps in one of their houses or in a restaurant. A trust fund is collected among mutually trusted friends, co-workers, and colleagues while they have fellowship, a party, or dinner together. The collected fund is used by one of them to pay for tuition, a wedding, a funeral, a new business, buying a house, and so on. The order of who uses the fund could be decided in relation to the priority needs of the members. If a person needs a big sum of money rather suddenly, *ge* is a way of arranging funding.

gingko biloba: Aging-control agent.

gi sung ie myun gam tchun 지성이면 감천 至誠感天: If one does one's best truly and sincerely, heaven will be impressed and will help the person to accomplish his or her wishes.

guer da non bori jaru 꿔다논 보리자루 (a borrowed bag of barley)**:** A person does not mix well with people and does not participate well in activities with people and this attitude might discourage others' enthusiasm as well.

gut 굿: A shamanistic ritual ceremony held to appease the spirits of ancestral or deceased family members, relatives, lovers, and others, and to ask them to grant wishes in a healing ceremony. A shaman, such as a spirit medium, officiates in the ceremony with music, dance, and conversation beyond time and space.

han 한 恨: regrets and resentments.

hanul gua dang i dul uh gin da 하늘과 땅이 떨어진다 (The earth and the sky are falling down): A sudden, extraordinarily chaotic, shocking crisis.

hanyak 한약 韓藥: Korean traditional medicine or herb medicine.

hon bea baek san 혼비 백산 魂飛魄散: The soul escapes from the body in an extraordinary, astonishing, or crisis situation.

hwabyung 화병 火病: Anger illness.

hwapoori 화 푸리: One becomes irritable or usually blames others for one's own mishaps to alleviate one's anger. Ways of releasing anger or frustration by blaming others or acting out.

hyun mo yang chuh 현모 양처 賢母良妻: A wise mother and a good wife.

jaab a muck da 잡아먹다: Kill and eat someone up.

jogwanggichur 조강지처 糟糠之妻: A man's formal wife, who patiently and quietly endures all pains, trials, and tribulations in marriage, usually related to unfair treatment by her unfaithful husband and his family members. At the end, her husband and his family especially recognize her as the one and only triumphant, honored, and proud wife, a *jogwang gichur*, usually among many wives.

jukgi mot hae suh saanda 죽지못해서 산다: Literally, a person who lives only because he or she cannot let himself or herself die. The real meaning is that one barely lives due to being unable to avoid extreme hardships.

kaji maneun namu param chalnal upda

가지 많은 나무 바람잘날 없다: A tree with many branches will not have moments of stillness undisturbed by the blowing wind. There is always something to do or problems to solve.

kimchi 김치: Vegetables such as cabbage and radishes that have been preserved with salt, garlic, and hot pepper.

kyung 경 經: A selected portion of Buddhist scriptures.

maum merk da 마음 먹다: To be determined, to make up one's mind, or to become one in body and mind.

maum ul pun da 마음을 푼다: Literally, loosening or unknotting emotions and a distressed mind. It means making oneself or someone else feel free from emotional distress, tension, conflicts, worries, frustration, or anger.

mert yt gae sal da 멋있게 산다: To be happy, not depressed; to live fully and meaningfully with style and vision.

nae sak ahn ha da 내색안 한다 (not showing inner colors): One does not share or publicize one's inner feelings or thinking, which could involve a stigmatized illness, secrets, inner conflicts, worries, hatred, resentment, regret, or something wonderful.

nammihoranggaenggyo: A religion related to Buddhism.

na nun bok i up nun sa ram iya 나는 복이 없는 사람이야: Happiness does not come to me as I deserve or wish.

nucduri 넉두리: Continuing to hold a grudge and complain.

oe yu na gang 외유내강 外柔內剛: Having a strongly and strictly disciplined inner self, being carefree and generous, and outwardly understanding others.

o nun chong i it ser ya ga nun chong do it da

오는 정이 있어야 가는정도 있다: If one cares for another person, the other will also care for that person in return and have mutual affection.

param pin da or **param pium** 바람피운다 (stir wind): Usually an unapproved relationship between a man and a woman, or extramarital affairs.

pung 풍 風: Literally, the wind. A broad Korean traditional and popular medical term indicating an idiosyncratic physical syndrome, usually with the sudden onset of a stroke, toothache with edema, erysipelas, or allergic reactions to foods.

sang byung 생병 生病: Literally, a live disease. The real meaning is to create illnesses unnecessarily due to lack of broad understanding of human nature and wisely regulating one's life.

shingyung 신경 神經: Literally and physically, it means nerves. Cognitively and emotionally, it means the mind, emotion, soul, distress, agony, or worry.

shingyungguamin 신경과민 神經過敏: Overly sensitive nerves. It is similar to *shingyungshayak* (neuralgia). However, it refers more to worrying, being irritable and restless, and intense concentration on problem solving, than to physical symptoms. *Shingyungguamin* seems to be related more to mental, emotional, and cognitive distress, while *shingyungshayak* tends to be the involvement of physical weakness as well as mental weakness due to *shingyungguamin*. Thus, *shingyungshayak* is the end product of *shingyungguamin*. It refers to someone who worries too much and is neurotic, nervous, or restless. Sometimes the person is excessively concerned with how others think of him or her.

shingyungjil 신경질 神經질: One behaves in a frustrated, angry, restless, or irritable manner. One may become bodily weakened or threatening toward others.

shingyung seun da 신경 쓴다: A state in which one thinks intensely to come up with solutions, or an individual is being bothered by anger, emotional distress, conflicts, stress, or worries.

shingyungshayak 신경쇠약 神經衰弱: Neurasthenia (see also *shingyungguamin*).

shingyungtong 신경통 神經痛: Literally, nerve pains. It usually indicates severe physical pains, aches, or pins and needles, usually on the shoulders, arms, back, thighs, legs, or buttocks, similar to neuralgia.

sokbyung 속병: Literally, inner illness. It can include chronic heartburn and indigestion, sometimes with stomach gas, originating from emotional distress and worries. It also means chronic emotional distress.

sok eul suk da 속이 썩다: Literally, "My inside is being rotten." One is angry, irritable, worried, or distressed.

sok i sang ha da 속이 상하다: Being injured inside. The emotional state of having anger, conflicts, jealousy, and resentment.

sooshin 수신 修身: Body training.

tae kwon do 태권도: Korean martial arts.

Tao 도 道: The way of conduct. A wise, pure, understanding, forgiving, open, deep, vast, dignified, and visionary way of living. Virtuous conduct as conceived by Confucians and Taoists. It is related to self-cultivation.

tchang 창: Koreans sing with thirty-six "colors" (types or kinds) of voice, which can be expressed as winding, pushing, stamping, knitting, cutting, sprinkling, or pressing, in mainly strenuous ways of vocalizing, to express various cognitive and emotional states.

ui chir jeung 의처증 疑妻症: A syndrome related to suspicion about a wife's chastity.

woohwangchungshimhwan 우황청심환 牛黃淸心丸: A medicinal tablet made of cow gallbladder and from other animal, herbal, and mineral elements for cooling the heart. It is a remedy for acute, life-threatening symptoms such as cardiorespiratory trouble, hypertension, seizure, or stroke. It is also taken as a tonic.

yin nae sim 인내심 忍耐心: Patience.

yshim junshim 이심전심 以心傳心: Insight, intuition, or knowing another's wishes or conditions through empathy or sympathy, without actually speaking about it.

Bibliography

American Psychiatric Association. 1980. *Diagnostic and Statistical Manual of Mental Disorders,* Third Edition. (DSM-III). Washington, DC: American Psychiatric Association.

American Psychiatric Association. 1987. *Diagnostic and Statistical Manual of Mental Disorders,* Third Edition, Revised. Washington, DC: American Psychiatric Association.

Angel, R. and P. Thoits. 1987. The impact of culture on the cognitive structure of illness. *Culture, Medicine and Psychiatry,* 11(4): 465-494.

Baik, S.C. 1984. The meaning of psychotherapy and its application in Korean society. *Korean Society and Culture,* 4: 273-313. Monograph Series 84-11. Sung Nam: Hanguk Jung Shin Mun Wha Research Institute.

Beck, A. 1976. *Cognitive Therapy and Emotional Disorders.* New York: International Universities Press.

Blatt, S.J. and D.C. Zuroff. 1992. Interpersonal relatedness and self-definition: Two prototypes for depression. *Clinical Psychology Review,* 12(5): 527-562.

Brody, H. 1987. *Stories of Sickness.* New Haven: Yale University Press.

Brown, G.W. and T. Harris. 1978. *Social Origins of Depression.* London: Free Press.

Bruner, J. 1986. *Actual Minds, Possible Worlds.* Cambridge, MA: Harvard University Press.

Burnside, I. 1994. Reminiscence group therapy. In I. Burnside and M.G. Schmidt, eds., *Working with Older Adults: Group Process and Techniques,* Third Edition. Boston: Jones and Bartlett Publishers, pp. 163-178.

Chang, S. 1996. Gut and psychodramatic treatment of death and bereavement. *Association of Korean American Psychiatrists Newsletter,* 7(3): 4-11.

Cheung, F.M., B.W. Law, and E. Waldmann. 1981. Somatization among Chinese depressives in general practice. *International Journal of Psychiatry in Medicine,* 10(4): 361-374.

Chin, L.C. 1993. Toward a psychology of difference: Psychotherapy for a culturally diverse population. In J.L. Chin, V. DeLa Cancela, and Y.M. Jenkins, eds., *Diversity in Psychotherapy: The Politics of Race, Ethnicity, and Gender.* London: Praeger, pp. 69-92.

Choi, J.S. 1964. Traditional values in Korean family. *Journal of Asiatic Studies,* 7(2): 43-47.

Choi, Y.D. 1995. *Bob Pur* (Serve Rice) II. Seoul: Dong-A Newspaper Company.

Chung, C.H. 1995. *Hanguk Chun Tong Sa Hoi ui Chung Shin Mun Hwa Gu Cho Yang Sang.* (The Pattern of Ethos in Traditional Korea: A Cross-Cultural Study of Value Orientation Through Examination of Proverbs.) Seoul: Korea University Press.

Clark, E.B. 1995. The sacred rights of the weak: Pain, sympathy, and the culture of individual rights in antebellum America. *The Journal of American History*, 82(2): 463-493.

Cohler, B. 1982. Personal narrative and the life course. In P. Balte and O. Brim, eds., *Life-Span Development and Behavior, Vol. 4*. New York: Academic Press, pp. 206-241.

Coles, R. and J.H. Coles. 1978. *Women of Crisis: Lives of Struggle and Hope*. Radcliffe Biography Series. New York: Delacorte Press.

Comfort Women Research Committee. 1995. *Jungguk eui ro guel yui gan Chosunyin Gun Weeahnbudeul.* (Korean Military Comfort Women, Who Were Taken to China.) Seoul: Han Wool (in Korean).

Cook, E.A. 1988. The effect of reminiscence group therapy on depressed institutionalized elders. Unpublished doctoral dissertation. Austin, TX: School of Nursing, the University of Texas.

Coryell, W., J. Endicott, G. Winokur, H. Akiskal, D. Solomon, A. Leon, T. Mueller, and T. Skea. 1995. Characteristics and significance of untreated major depressive disorder. *American Journal of Psychiatry*, 152(8): 1124-1129.

Dallet, C. 1954. *Traditional Korea*. New Haven: Human Relations Area Files (English Translation). (Originally published as *Choson Kyohoesa*. N.-J. Lee and J. Yoon [trans.], Korean translation, 1947, Seoul: Dae Sung Publishing, 1947.

Depner, C.E. and B. Ingersoll-Dayton. 1985. Conjugal social support: Patterns in later life. *Journal of Gerontology*, 40(6): 761-766.

Eckert, C.J., K.-B. Lee, Y.I. Lew, M. Robinson, and E.W. Wagner. 1990. *Korea Old and New: A History*. Seoul: Ilchokak.

Epstein, S.J. 1995. Wanderers in the wilderness: Image of America in Ch'oe In-Ho's Kipko Pu'urun Pam. *Korea Journal*, 35(4): 72-79.

Escobar, J.I., A. Burnam, M. Karno, A. Forsythe, and J.M. Golding. 1987. Somatization in the community. *Archives of General Psychiatry*, 44(8): 713-718.

Ferrara, K.W. 1994. *Therapeutic Ways with Words*. Oxford, UK: Oxford University Press.

Finch, J. 1989. *Family Obligations and Social Change*. Oxford, UK: Polity Press.

Finkler, K. 1994. *Woman in Pain: Gender and Morbidity in Mexico*. Philadelphia: University of Pennsylvania Press.

Gee, J. 1985. The narrativization of experience in the oral style. *Journal of Education*, 167(1): 9-35.

Gibran, K. 1989. *The Prophet*. New York: Alfred A. Knopf.

Good, B.J. 1977. The heart of what's the matter: The semantics of illness in Iran. *Culture, Medicine and Psychiatry*, 1(1): 25-58.

Good, B.J. and M.D. Good. 1981. The meaning of symptoms: A cultural hermeneutic model for clinical practice. In L. Eisenberg and A. Kleinman, eds., *The Relevance of Social Science for Medicine*. Boston: D. Reidel Publishing Co., pp. 165-196.

Good, B.J., M.D. Good, and R. Moradi. 1985. The interpretation of Iranian depressive illness and dysphoric affects. In A. Kleinman and B.J. Good, eds., *Culture and Depression.* Berkeley: University of California Press, pp. 369-428.

Gordon, J.S. 1996. *Manifesto for a New Medicine.* New York: Addison-Wesley.

Ha, H.T. 1964. *Maxims and Proverbs of Old Korea.* Korean Cultural Series Vol. VII. Seoul: Yonsei University Press.

Hahn, D.S. Psychiatry in Seoul, Korea. In *Collection of Scientific Papers in Commemoration of the Sixtieth Birthday on March 17, 1965 of Prof. Choo-Wan Myung, M.D.* Seoul: Department of Neuropsychiatry College of Medicine, Seoul National University, Korea, 1: pp. 68-75.

Harvey, Y.K. 1979. *Six Korean Women: The Socialization of Shamans.* St. Paul, MN: West Publishing Co.

Helgeson, V.S. 1994. Relation of agency and communion to well-being: Evidence and potential explanations. *Psychology Bulletin,* 116(3): 412-428.

Janelli, R.L. and D.Y. Janelli. 1982. *Ancestor Worship and Korean Society.* Stanford, CA: Stanford University Press.

Kalish, R.A. 1968. Suicide: An ethnic comparison in Hawaii. *Bulletin of Suicidology,* (4): 37-43.

Kang, H.S. 1981. *Dong Yang Eui Hak Gae Ron.* (Comprehensive Asian Medical Theory and Practice.) Seoul: Go Mun Sa Publishers.

Katon, W., A. Kleinman, and G. Rosen. 1982. Depression and somatization: A review, parts I and II. *American Journal of Medicine,* 72(1): 127-135, (2): 241-247.

Kim, B.I. 1996. Modern Korean literature: Its past, present and future. *Koreana,* 10(2): 4-9.

Kim, B.S. 1980. The functions of conflict in the construction of Korean-American communities. In B.S. Kim and S.H. Lee, eds. *The Korean Immigrant in America.* Montclair: AKCS in North America, Inc., pp. 147-162.

Kim, J.H. 1975. *Myung Shim Bo Gam.* (Treasured Collection of Moral Lessons.) Seoul: Myung Mun Sa.

Kim, J.W. 1998. Sadness governs anger. *The Korean Weekly Washington,* January 15, no. 345, p. 37.

Kim, K. 1997. Clinical study of primary depressive symptom. Part III: A cross-cultural comparison: Korea, England, United States and India. *Neuropsychiatry (Journal of Korean Neuropsychiatric Association),* 16(1): 53-60.

Kim, K.-I. 1991. *Hanguk Juntong Munhwa Eui Jungshin bunsuk: Shinhwa, Musok Gue Ri Go Jonggyo Chehum* (Psychoanalytic Interpretation of Korean Traditional Culture: Myth, Shamanism, and Religious Experiences). Seoul: Kyomunsa (in Korean).

Kim, K.I. and B.Y. Rhi. 1976. A review of Korean cultural psychiatry. *Transcultural Psychiatric Research Review,* 13(October): 101-114.

Kim, K.-I., D. Li, Z. Jiang, X. Cui, L. Lin, J.J. Kang, K.K. Park, E. (K.) K. Chung, and C.K. Kim. 1993. Schizophrenic delusions among Koreans, Korean-Chinese, and Chinese: Transcultural Chinese delusions of religious or supernatural matters. *The International Journal of Social Psychiatry,* 39(3): 190-199.

Kim, L. 1991. Korean ethos: Concept of Jeong, Haan and others. A paper presented at the scientific meeting of Pacific Rim College of Psychiatrists, Los Angeles, CA. October 17-20.

Kim, M.H. 1996. Changing relationships between daughters-in-law and mothers-in-law in urban South Korea. *Anthropology Quarterly,* 69(4): 179-192.

Kirmayer, L.J. 1989. Cultural variations in the response to psychiatric disorders and emotional distress. *Social Science and Medicine,* 29(3): 327-339.

Kleinman, A. 1980. *Patients and Healers in the Context of Culture.* Berkeley: University of California.

Kleinman, A. 1982. Neurasthenia and depression: A study of somatization and culture in China. *Culture, Medicine and Psychiatry,* 6(2): 117-190.

Kleinman, A. 1986. *Social Origins of Distress and Disease.* New Haven: Yale University Press.

Kleinman, A. 1995. *Writing at the Margin: Discourse Between Anthropology and Medicine.* Berkeley: University of California Press.

Kleinman, A. and B. Good. 1985. Introduction: Culture and depression. In A. Kleinman and B. Good, eds., *Culture and Depression.* Berkeley: University of California Press, pp. 1-33.

Kleinman, A. and J. Kleinman. 1985. Somatization: The interconnections in Chinese society among culture, depressive experiences, and the meanings of pain. In A. Kleinman and B. Good, eds., *Culture and Depression.* Berkeley: University of California Press, pp. 429-489

Koenig, H.G., L.K. George, and I.C. Siegler. 1988. The use of religion and other emotion-regulating coping strategies among older adults. *The Gerontologist,* 28(3): 303-310.

Koh, H.C. 1983. Korean women, conflict, and change: An approach to development planning. In L. Kendall and M. Peterson, eds., *Korean Women: View from the Inner Room.* New Haven: East Rock Press, pp. 159-175.

Korean Dictionary. 1995. Third Edition. Seoul: Min Jung Suh Rim.

Korea Survey Gallup Polls. 1990. *Life Style and Value System of the Aged in Korea.* Seoul: Korea Survey Gallup.

Korte, A.O. 1979. Interpretive Research Approaches and the Mexicano Elders. In E.P. Stanford, ed., *Minority Aging Research: Old Issues, New Approaches.* San Diego: San Diego State University, pp. 105-114.

Kuo, W.H. 1984. Prevalence of depression among Asian-Americans. *Journal of Nervous and Mental Disease,* 172(8): 449-457.

Kuo, W.H. and Y.M. Tsai. 1986. Social networking, hardiness, and immigrants' mental health. *Journal of Health Social Behavior,* 27(2): 133-149.

Lee, H. 1996. *Still Life with Rice: A Young American Woman Discovers the Life and Legacy of Her Korean Grandmother.* New York: Scribners.

Lee, J.G. 1997. I give the Goliath's republic to my son San Ha. *Mal* (A Journal in Korean), 133: 202-205.

Lee, K.-B. 1984. *A New History of Korea*. Translated by E.W. Wagner with E.J. Shultz. Seoul: Ilchokak.

Lee, K.T. 1977. *Hanguk In eu Eusik Gujo* (The Frame of Mind of Koreans). Seoul: Mun Ri Sa (in Korean).

Lee, K.T. 1987. Han puri mu. (Han unknotting dance.) *Cho Sun Newspaper.* July 11, p .2 (in Korean, U.S. Edition).

Lee, K.T. 1992. *Korean Studies of Tears*. Seoul: Kirinwon (in Korean).

Lee, M.H., H.Y. Lee, S.K. Min, K.H. Kim, S.Y. Kim, D.H. Song, J.H. Shin, M.H. Park, A. Bae, and K.Y. Sung. 1986. Development of Korean version of the NIMH Diagnostic Interview Schedule and its validity test—Kangwha Psychiatric Epidemiological Survey (I). *Neuropsychiatry,* 25(2): 300-313.

Lee, O.Y. 1967. *In This Earth and in That Wind: This is Korea*. Translated by D.I. Steinberg. Seoul: Hollym Corp.

Lee, Seung Hyun. 1990. *Dan Hak.* (Study of Truth. Theory and Practice.) Seoul: Doe Suh Chul Paan Yu Riem.

Lee, Si Hyung. 1977. Psychogenic pain: Its meaning and therapy. *Human Sciences,* 1(6): 39(344)-43(447) (In Korean.)

Lee, Si Hyung. 1987. *Let Us Live with Bluffness and Confidence.* Seoul: Jipyunjun.

Lin, K.-M. 1983. *Hwabyung:* A Korean culture-bound syndrome? *American Journal of Psychiatry,* 140(1): 105-107.

Luborsky, M.R. 1995. Questioning the allure of aging and health for medical anthropology. *Medical Anthropology Quarterly,* 9(2): 277-283.

Lutz, C. 1985. Depression and the translation of emotional worlds. In A. Kleinman and B. Good, eds., *Culture and Depression: Studies in the Anthropology and Cross-Cultural Psychiatry of Affect and Disorder.* Berkeley: University of California Press, pp. 63-100.

Mackenzie, A.E. and E. Holroyd. 1995. An exploration of carers' perceptions of care giving and caring in Chinese families. *International Journal of Nursing Studies,* 33(1): 1-12.

Marsella, A.J. and V.A. Kameoka. 1989. Ethnocultural issues in the assessment of psychopathology. In S. Wetzler, ed., *Measuring Mental Illness: Psychometric Assessment Clinicians,* Washington, DC: American Psychiatric Press, pp. 229-256.

Murphy, J.E. 1982. Social origins of depression in old age. *The British Journal of Psychiatry,* 141(August): 135-142.

Ngan, R. and I.C.K. Chang. 1992. The caring dilemma, stress and needs of carers for the Chinese frail elderly. *Hong Kong Journal of Gerontology,* 6(2): 34-41.

Nolen-Hoeksema, S. 1987. Sex differences in unipolar depression: Evidence and theory. *Psychological Bulletin,* 101(2): 259-282.

Ohnuki-Tierney, E. 1984. *Illness and Culture in Contemporary Japan*. New York: Cambridge University Press.

Pang, K.Y.C. 1991. *Korean Elderly Women in America: Everyday Life, Health, and Illness*. New York: AMS Press, Inc.

Pang, K.Y.C. 1998. Symptoms of depression in elderly Korean immigrants: Narration and the healing process. *Culture, Medicine, and Psychiatry,* 22(1): 93-122.

Pang, K.Y.C. 1995. A cross-cultural understanding of depression among elderly Korean immigrants: Prevalence, symptoms, and diagnosis. *Clinical Gerontologist,* 15(4): 3-20.

Pang, K.Y.C. 1996. Self-care in elderly Korean immigrants. *Journal of Cross-Cultural Gerontology,* 11(3): 229-254.

Park, K.R. 1990. Alternative thinking. In *Won Ju Correspondence.* Fifth Edition. Seoul: Ji Sik San Uph Sa, p. 99.

Park, S.B. 1995. Buddhist ethics in contemporary Korea. *Korean Culture,* 16(3): 20-25.

Park, W.-S. 1995. *Ger San ie Jungmal Kerki It Sur Cil Ka?* (Was the Mountain Really There?) Seoul: Ung Chin Printing Co.

Park, W.-S. 1996. In the realm of the Buddha. Translated by B. Fulton and J.C. Fulton. *Koreana,* 10(2): 81-91.

Rhi, B.Y. 1980. *Shamanism gua Shaman: Hanguk Sasang eui Wontien* (Shamanism and Shaman: The Origin of Korean Ethos). Seoul: Bak Young Sa (in Korean).

Rhi, B.Y. 1983. *Hangukin of Yunriguan* (Korean Ethos). Seoul: Korean Cultural Research Center (in Korean).

Rhi, B.Y. 1986. Hanguk eu Yugyo uwa Chungshin Gungang: *Yugyogurn Gazok eu Munhwa Simrijuk Guzo, Guague uwa Mirae.* (Confucianism and Mental Health in Korea: The Psycho-Cultural Dynamics of the Confucian Family, Past and Present.) Seoul: International Cultural Society of Korea, pp. 249-276 (in Korean).

Riesman, D. 1969. *The Lonely Crowd: A Study of the Changing American Character.* New Haven, CT: Yale University Press.

Robins, L.N., J.E. Helzer, J. Croughan, and K.S. Ratcliff. 1981. National Institute of Mental Health Diagnostic Interview Schedule: Its history, characteristics, and validity. *Archives of General Psychiatry,* 38(4): 381-389.

Sakauye, K.M., F.M. Baker, R.C. Chacko, R.G. Jimenez, H.W. Nickens, and J.W. Thompson. 1994. *Ethnic Minority Elderly. A Task Force Report of the American Psychiatric Association.* Washington, DC: American Psychiatric Association.

Shin, J.G.. 1983. *Buddhism and Medicine.* Seoul: Dong Guk University Press.

Shore, B. 1997. Keeping the conversation going: An interview with Jerome Bruner. *Ethos,* 25(1): 7-62.

Silverman, C. 1968. *The Epidemiology of Depression.* Baltimore: Johns Hopkins University Press.

Sim, J.L. 1995. The wisdom of delivering one's soul from suffering. *Philosophy and Reality,* 24: 208-217 (in Korean).

Sirkin, M.G. 1970. Household surveys with multiplicity. *Journal of American Statistical Association,* 65: 257.

Smith, B. 1980. Narrative versions, narrative theories. *Critical Inquiry,* 7(1): 212-236.

Suzuki, H. 1996. Life, Death, and Eternity. Speech at The Lady of Mercy Church, Potomac, Maryland, on Thursday, July 18.

Tower, R.B. and S.V. Kasl. 1996. Gender, marital closeness, and depressive symptoms in elderly couples. *Journal of Gerontology: Psychological Sciences,* 51B(3): 115-129.

Unschuld, P. 1985. *Medicine in China: A History of Ideas.* Berkeley: University of California Press.

U.S. Bureau of the Census. 1990. *Census of Population.* Washington, DC: United States Department of Commerce.

Weil, A. 1995. *Spontaneous Healing.* New York: Random House.

Yi, H.-D. 1973. Développement de la notion de piété filiale en Corée. *Revue de Corée,* 5(2): 5-23.

Yu, J.-H. 1997. Crisp portrayals of bleak lives Su, Chung-in. Koreana. *Korean Art & Culture.* 11 (2): 90-92.

Yun, H. 1976. The Korean personality and treatment considerations. *Social Casework,* 57(3): 173-178.

Index